WINGS OF HOME SCIENCE

WINGS OF HOME SCIENCE

Ms. Maimun Nisha

Publications

KALPAZ PUBLICATIONS

Delhi - 110052

Wings of Home Science

ISBN : 81-7835-504-3

Rs. 750

Published in 2006 in India by
Kalpaz Publications
C-30, Satyawati Nagar,
Delhi - 110052
e-mail : kalpaz@hotmail.com

Laser Typesetting at : Master Computer, Delhi
Printed at : Salasar Imaging System, Delhi

Contents

SECTION-C : CHILD PSYCHOLOGY

SECTION D : HOME SCIENCE

Preface

It is a great pleasure to note that *Wings of Home Science* will be popular among the students in recent future.

This book closely follows the syllabus prescribed by the universities in India department of home science.

This book covers the syllabus of Indian university of home science which represent the four different division of home science subject which reflect by part A, B, C and D. Part A represent the food and nutrition side where as Part B represent child development and study. Part C covers the child psychology portion where as Part D reflect the Home Science and its application.

This book represents, in Part A, about the food and nutrition, nutrients and its function, type, classification and their contribution, energy, meal planning, food preservation, food groups, food adulteration, food preparation, storage of food, health, water, food hygiene, and food borne illness. In Part B, the writer describe about the developmental chart of children, feeding of the baby, prenatal care, intra-natal care, sex development of the child, play development, baby care, growth and development, immunization for baby and childhood problems. Part C covers child psychology, physical growth, sensory motor growth, cognitive growth, emotional growth, individual difference, personality, learning process, language growth and social growth of the child. Part D represent the Home Science and its application.

The book title shows it is a primary book of home science for the students of university / classes as well as undergraduate/classes.

This book is helpful them and covers the all chapters and courses of the universities, department Home Science, Psychology, Child Development, Child Care and others.

This book is beneficent to that student who want to established their carrier in Home Science.

This book also helpful the student who will research in Home Science and Child Study in future.

This book should be of use not only the students as a textbook but also to the guide for teacher of Home Science departments.

I feel very happy in presenting the book to all universities students of Home Science, Child Study, Psychology and other subjects. All the chapters are uptodate study.

The author likes this opportunity to thank her well wishers and her publisher.

Maimun Nisha

SECTION-A
FOOD AND NUTRITION

1

Food and Nutrition

Definition of Food

Food is any substance normally eaten or drunk by living organisms. The term food also includes liquid drinks. Food is the main source of energy and of nutrition for animals, and is usually of animal or plant origin.

Definition of Nutrition

Nutrition is the study of the relationship between diet and states of health and disease. The vast majority of matter and energy required by an animal is obtained through the diet. Obviously, if an animal does not ingest any food or drink, it will not be able to meet its needs for matter or energy and will eventually die. Between the extremes of optimal health and death from starvation, there are an array of disease states that can be caused or alleviated by changes in diet. For example, a particular diet may meet an organism's requirements energy and protein, but lack a particular substance that the animal requires, such as Vitamin C. Without Vitamin C, the organism will eventually suffer from some variety of sub-optimal health, such as scurvy. In other cases, excesses or imbalances in the diet can have have negative impacts on health, resulting in disease states such as obesity or osteoporosis. Finally, substances such as lead may be ingested by an organism have specific toxic effects.

Overview of Nutrition

Nutrition can be defined as the study of foods and how foodstuffs affect health and biological function of the organism. The term nutrients refer to those chemical substances in foods that are required in the diet for survival and well being of the organism. This course will focus on the chemical composition and function of nutrients that is carbohydrates, fats (lipids), proteins, vitamins and minerals and water.

Organisms are composed of 'cells' that are the functioning units of the body. Cells are said to be self-replenishing that is when components are broken down those components can be rebuilt from substances provided in the diet. Cells are also said to be energy-converting units that is they take one form of energy and convert it into chemical energy used in the cell for rebuilding new components or for movement. Thus nutrients play a role in providing or using raw materials to rebuild body components and for providing energy. *Nutrition* then refers to the chemical components that are required in the diet for the organism to function normally. *Metabolism* refers to the chemical processes involved in the use of nutrients. Our approach to the topic of nutrition can be said to have a biochemical focus at a level that can be understood by those who do not have a background in chemistry.

The chemical composition and function of nutrients, participants are often surprised at the amount of chemistry that is part of the topic of 'nutrition'. For understanding nutrition one needs to know the fundamental building block of the large molecules (biomacromolecules) that are nutrients. For example sugars are the building blocks of many complex carbohydrates, amino acids are the building units for proteins and fatty acids are the main components of lipids (fats). When the biomacromolecules are ingested, they must be broken down (hydrolyzed) to their component units in order to be absorbed for use by the body. For example cellulose and starch are both carbohydrates and each consisting only of the simple sugar glucose as the building unit. The ability of the human being to digest and utilize the glucose in starch, but not in cellulose is a function of how the building blocks are connected and what enzymes are available for digestion.

Defining terms is a key to understanding the facts and concepts that will be presented. The following is a list of terms often seen in the press or on food labels: Low carbohydrates, unsaturated fats, saturated fats, high protein, and vitamin enriched. Without understanding definitions and the chemical nature of the substances, the significance of terms can be vague. For example, the term carbohydrate applies to sugars (table sugar or sucrose) as well as to starch and fibers. Sucrose is composed of two simple sugars; glucose and fructose linked together. Starch consists of hundreds of glucose units linked together. The body can only absorb simple sugars from the digestive tract hence sucrose or starch must be digested to the component simple sugars. Fiber on the other hand is not digested and cannot be absorbed hence its function as 'bulk'. In the current 'low carbohydrates' fad, many food products contain *sugar alcohols*. Technically, by definition, sugar alcohols are not carbohydrates. Sugar alcohols are poorly absorbed across the intestine and therefore remain in the intestine until excreted. As we shall see, substances that are not absorbed from the intestine remain there with resulting consequences that will be discussed tactfully.

Once nutrients are absorbed across the intestine, the fate of those substances involves events related to metabolism, the chemical conversion of those substances. The conversion of foodstuffs to energy is perhaps one of the most complex topics to be discussed. The idea is that nutrients like glucose contain 'potential energy'. The body converts (burns or oxidizes) glucose to carbon dioxide and water and releases energy in the form that is usable for biological processes. The energy content of foodstuffs is given in calories and we will see that calories do count in terms of maintaining body weight.

The epidemic of obesity is a topic that is prevalent in the news media and of great public health concern. One of the culprits is alleged to be High Fructose Corn Syrup (HFCS) that is used to sweeten desserts, candy and beverages. The consumption of large amounts of HFCS provides the body with a large amount of well absorbed simple sugar and floods the body with a nutrient that can be readily turned in to 'fat'. One objective of this course is to provide the participants with information on the chemical nature of nutrients with an understanding of the basic principles of metabolism that will be of value in making dietary choices.

The course will include a discussion of a number of hormones. Many of those chemical messengers play a role in the use or storage of nutrients. The hormones *insulin* and *glucagons* play opposing roles in the storage and use of glucose. The news media have presented stories on the 'scandals' related to the use of *steroids* by professional as well as high school athletes. There are a number of different classes of steroid hormones, those that act as *protein anabolic steroids* act to increase the musculature of the individual taking those steroids. Thyroid hormones influence the rate of metabolism of an individual and thyroid gland activity may need to be evaluated by overweight individuals seeking to loose weight.

Functions of Food

Food serves three functions in most living organisms. First, it provides materials that are metabolized either by oxidative or by fermentative processes to supply the energy required for the absorption and translocation of nutrients, for the synthesis of cell materials, for motility and locomotion, for excretion of waste products, and for all other activities.

Nutrients

Nutrients are chemical elements and compounds found in the environment that plants and animals need to grow and survive. For water-quality investigations the various forms of nitrogen and phosphorus are the nutrients of interest. The forms include nitrate, nitrite, ammonia, organic nitrogen (in the form of plant material or other organic compounds), and phosphates (orthophosphate and others). Nitrate is the most common form of nitrogen and phosphates are the most common forms of phosphorus found in natural waters. High concentrations of nutrients in water bodies can potentially cause eutrophication and hypoxia.

To function, the human body must have nutrients. The nutrients known to be essential for human beings are proteins, carbohydrates, fats and oils, minerals, vitamins and water.

Sources and the Function of Nutrients

Calories

Calories are needed to provide energy so the body functions properly. The number of calories in a food depends on the amount of energy the food provides. The number of calories a person needs depends on age, height, weight, gender, and activity level. People who consume more calories than they burn off in normal daily activity or during exercise are more likely to be overweight.

Fat:	1 gram	=	9 calories
Protein:	1 gram	=	4 calories
Carbohydrates:	1gram	=	4 calories
Alcohol:	1 gram	=	7 calories

Fat

Fat should account for 30 per cent or less of the calories consumed daily, with saturated fats accounting for no more than 10 per cent of the total fat intake. Fats are a concentrated form of energy which help maintain body temperature, and protect body tissues and organs. Fat also plays an essential role in carrying the four fat-soluble Vitamins A, D, E and K.

Excess calories from protein and carbohydrates are converted to and stored as fat. Even if you are eating mostly "fat free" foods, excess consumption will result in additional body fat. Fat calories in food are readily stored, while it takes energy to transform protein and carbohydrates to body fat. The only proven way to reduce body fat is to burn more calories than one consumes.

Saturated Fat

- tends to increase blood cholesterol levels. Most saturated fats tend to be solid at room temperature, with the exception of tropical oils.

- found mostly in meat and dairy products, as well as some vegetable oils, such as coconut and palm oils (tropical oils). Butter is high in saturated fat, while margarine tends to have more unsaturated fat.

Polyunsaturated Fat

- tends to lower blood cholesterol levels.

- found mostly in plant sources (safflower, sunflower, soybean, corn, cottonseed).

Monounsaturated Fat

- tends to lower LDL cholesterol (the "bad" cholesterol).
- found in both plant and animal products, such as olive oil, canola oil, peanut oil, and in some plant foods such as avocado.

Cholestrol

Chloestrol intake should not exceed 300 milligrams a day. Individuals differ on their absorption of dietary cholesterol, what is important is one's level of blood cholesterol. High blood cholesterol has been linked to the occurrence of atherosclerosis. Atherosclerosis is a buildup of fatty deposits in the coronary arteries and other blood vessels, and is a leading cause of heart attacks.

Dietary cholesterol is only found in foods from *animal* sources, including meat, fish, milk, eggs, cheese and butter. You may have heard the terms HDL and LDL discussed in relation to blood cholesterol and heart disease. HDL and LDL are lipoproteins, substances found in the bloodstream that transport cholesterol and triglycerides in the body.

- HDLs help remove cholesterol from the blood, protecting you from heart disease (atherosclerosis).
- LDLs are thought to deposit cholesterol in artery walls, increasing your risk of heart disease (atherosclerosis). Most abundant type, LDL carries approximately 65% of the total circulating cholesterol. High levels of LDL are associated with atherosclerosis.

Carbohydrates

Carbohydrates are a major source of energy and should account for 50 per cent to 60 per cent of calories consumed each day.

Sugars:

- Monosaccharides and disaccharides.
- found in fruits (sucrose, glucose, fructose, pentose), milk (lactose), and softdrinks and sweets.

Complex:

- Polysaccharides.

Carbohydrates:

- Found in whole grain cereals, flour, bread, rice, corn, oats, potatoes and legumes.

Dietary Fiber

Sources of fiber from highest to lowest are high fiber grain products, nuts, legumes (kidney, navy, black and pinto beans), vegetables, fruits, and refined grain products.

Soluble fiber:

- may help lower blood cholesterol by inhibiting digestion of fat and cholesterol; helps control blood sugar in people with diabetes.
- found in peas, beans, oats, barley, some fruits and vegetables (apples, oranges, carrots), and psyllium.

Insoluble fiber:

- helps prevent constipation, hemorrhoids, and diverticulosis.
- found in bran (wheat, oat, and rice), wheat germ, cauliflower, green beans, potatoes, celery.

Protein

Protein should account for 10 per cent to 20 per cent of the calories consumed each day. Protein is essential to the structure of red blood cells, for the proper functioning of antibodies resisting infection, for the regulation of enzymes and hormones, for growth, and for the repair of body tissue.

Amino acids are the building blocks of protein and are found in a variety of foods. Meat, milk, cheese, and egg are complete proteins that have all the essential amino acids. Other sources of protein include whole grains, rice, corn, beans, legumes, oatmeal, peas, and peanut butter. For those who do not eat meat, eggs, or dairy products, it is important to eat a variety of these other foods in order to get enough protein.

Vitamins and Minerals

Vitamins and minerals are required for the regulation of the body's metabolic functions, and are found naturally in the foods we eat. Many foods are fortified in order to provide additional nutrients, or to replace nutrients that may have been lost during the processing of the food. Most people are able to obtain satisfactory nutrition from the wide selection of foods available in the United States.

If a person is not able to eat a variety of foods from the basic food groups, then a vitamin and mineral supplement may be necessary. However, except for certain unusual health conditions, very few persons should need more than 100 per cent of the Recommended Daily Allowance for any single nutrient. Large doses of vitamin and mineral supplements can be harmful.

Vitamins come in two varieties: fat soluble and water-soluble. Fat-soluble vitamins can be stored in the body for long periods of time, while excess amounts of water-soluble vitamins are excreted in the urine.

Vitamin A • Needed for new cell growth,

healthy skin, hair, and tissues, and vision in dim light.

- *Sources*: Dark green and yellow vegetables and yellow fruits, such as broccoli spinach, turnip greens, carrots, squash, sweet potatoes, pumpkin, cantaloupe, and apricots, and in animal sources such as liver, milk, butter, cheese, and whole eggs.

Vitamin D

- Promotes absorption and use of calcium and phosphate for healthy bones and teeth.
- *Sources:* Milk (fortified), cheese, whole eggs, liver, salmon, and fortified margarine. The skin can synthesize Vitamin D if exposed to enough sunlight on a regular basis.

Vitamin E

- Protects red blood cells and helps prevent destruction of Vitamins A and C.
- *Sources:* Margarine and vegetable oil (soybean, corn, safflower, and cottonseed), wheat germ, green leafy vegetables.

Vitamin K

- Necessary for normal blood clotting and synthesis of proteins found in plasma, bone, and kidneys.
- *Sources:* Spinach, lettuce, kale, cabbage, cauliflower, wheat bran, organ meats, cereals, some fruits, meats, dairy products, eggs.

Vitamin C	• An antioxidant vitamin needed for the formation of collagen to hold the cells together and for healthy teeth, gums and blood vessels; improves iron absorption and resistance to infection. • *Sources:* Many fresh vegetables and fruits, such as broccoli, green and red peppers, collard greens, sprouts, cauliflower, lemon, cabbage, pineapples, strawberries, citrus fruits.
Thiamin (B1)	• Needed for energy metabolism and the proper function of the nervous system. • *Sources:* Whole grains, soybeans, peas, and liver, and kidney, lean cuts of pork, legumes, seeds, and nuts.
Riboflavin (B2)	• Needed for energy metabolism, building tissue, and helps maintain good vision. • *Sources:* Dairy products, lean meats, poultry, fish, grains, broccoli, turnip greens, asparagus, spinach, and enriched food products.
Niacin	• Needed for energy metabolism, proper digestion, and healthy nervous system. • *Sources:* Lean meats, liver, poultry, milk, canned salmon, leafy green vegetables.
Vitamin B6 (Pyridoxine)	• Needed for cell growth. • *Sources:* Chicken, fish, pork, liver, kidney, whole grains, nuts, and legumes.

Foliate (Folic acid)	• Promotes normal digestion; essential for development of red blood cells. • *Sources:* Liver, yeast, dark green leafy vegetables, legumes, and some fruits.
Vitamin B_{12}	• Needed for building proteins in the body, red blood cells, and normal function of nervous tissus. • *Sources*: Liver, kidney, yogurt, dairy products, fish, clams, oysters, nonfat dry milk, salmon, sardines.
Calcium	• Needed for healthy bones and teeth, normal blood clotting, and nervous system functioning. • *Sources*: Dairy products, broccoli, cabbage, kale, tofu, sardines and salmon.
Iron	• Needed for the formation of hemoglobin, which carries oxygen from the lungs to the body cells. • *Sources:* Meats, eggs, dark green leafy vegetables, legumes, whole grains and enriched food products.
Phosphorus	• Needed for healthy bones and teeth, energy metabolism, and acid base balance in the body. • *Sources:* Milk, grains, lean meats, food additives.
Magnesium	• Needed for healthy bones and teeth, proper nervous system functioning, and energy metabolism. • *Sources*: Dairy products, meat, fish, poultry, green vegetables, legumes.
Zinc	• Needed for cell reproduction, tissue growth and repair.

	• *Sources*: Meat, seafood, and liver, eggs, milk, whole-grain products.
Pantothenic Acid	• Needed for energy metabolism. • *Sources:* Egg yolk, liver, kidney, yeast, broccoli, lean beef, skim milk, sweet potatoes, molasses.
Copper	• Needed for synthesis of hemoglobin, proper iron metabolism, and maintenance of blood vessels. • *Sources:* Seafood, nuts, legumes, green leafy vegetables.
Manganese	• Needed for enzyme structure. • *Sources:* Whole grain products, fruits and vegetables, tea.

Water

In order to live, every cell in the body must be bathed in water. Water takes an active part in many chemical reactions and is needed to carry other nutrients, to regulate body temperature, and to help eliminate wastes. Water makes up about 60 per cent of an adult's body weight. Requirements for water are met in many ways. Most fruits are more than 90 per cent water.

Intracellular Function of Essential Nutrients

Nutrient deficiencies may be induced by a variety of conditions. With a functional deficiency, a nutrient may be present, but it may not be properly activated, it may not be appropriately localized, or it may not have sufficient cofactors to function at a normal level of activity. Underlying reasons for a functional nutrient deficiency include inefficiencies or deficiencies in the following:

- absorption by the gastrointestinal tract–intracellular activation.
- transport to the appropriate tissue–storage.
- transport through the cell membrane–concentration or activity of cofactors.
- presence of intracellular inhibitors–tissues with increased metabolic needs.

Thus, a functional deficiency includes anything that may reduce the concentration or the efficacy of a nutrient. No matter what the underlying cause, the result will be a defect in the biochemical pathways that depend upon the optimal function of that nutrient. A deficient or defective pathway may operate at a sub-optimal level for many months or even years before a clinical symptom may become apparent.

Nutrients May Enhance Immune Function in the Elderly

Many older adults have to deal with a host of medical issues that put them at risk for malnutrition, a condition that makes them more susceptible to infection. As the number of people over age 65 continues to grow, strategies to reduce this risk are under investigation. A recent article in *Clinical Infectious Diseases* summarizes current research into nutritional intervention as a way of boosting immune status and preventing infections in the elderly.

Immune Dysfunctions in the Elderly

Infection is a common problem among older Americans, who are 2 to 10 times more likely to die of infection than younger adults. An age-related decline in immune function probably contributes to that risk, as cells become less able to stimulate an adaptive immune response. Scientists are not yet sure to what degree nutrient deficiencies contribute to that deterioration, in part because there is not yet agreement on what levels of intake will insure adequate absorption. They are, however, taking a close look at how certain nutrients - including vitamin E and trace minerals zinc and selenium - affect infection rate in medically frail older adults.

Nutrition Supplement

That is it difficult to make specific recommendations concerning the benefit of vitamin and mineral supplements due to the diversity of study findings. He concludes, though, that there are enough data to support the use of a daily multivitamin that includes zinc (20 mg), selenium (100 micrograms), and Vitamin E (200 mg). In his opinion, supplements that provide these nutrients may reduce the rate of infections, along with the use of antibiotics, in older adults.

Nutrition supplements serve little purpose unless the underlying cause of malnutrition–be it chronic illness, poorly fitting dentures, depression, or medication-induced anorexia–is identified and treated. A new website sponsored by the American Academy of Family Physicians and the American, The site's key document, The Role of Nutrition in Chronic Disease Care outlines the nutritional management of chronic illnesses–including cancer, congestive heart failure, pneumonia, and dementia–that can put seniors at risk for malnutrition.

Several studies have shown that both zinc and selenium supplements may enhance immune function and reduce the risk of infection. There is some evidence that zinc, in combination with adequate protein and calories, can reduce the incidence of pressure ulcers in institutionalized adults. The author notes that zinc is often the nutrient of choice to promote wound healing, but zinc supplementation may be best suited to those who are malnourished, and likely zinc deficient.

Vitamin E, a potent antioxidant, has also been linked to improved immune response. Few studies, though, have demonstrated the ability of Vitamin E to affect clinical end points, such as fewer infections or less antibiotic use, in elderly patients. How much Vitamin E is needed to see an effect is still an issue. Researchers have been able to show improved immune response at doses ranging from 200 mg to 800 mg per day. Current U.S. dietary intake recommendations for Vitamin E, however, fall far below this level.

2
Protein

Proteins are made of amino acids, small units necessary for growth and tissue repair. Protein is the body's most plentiful substance except for water and, possibly, fat. Animal foods such as meat, fish, poultry, milk, and eggs are rich in protein. Good plant sources of protein are beans, peas, nuts, bread, and cereals.

Every single cell in your body is made up of protein. Hair and fingernails consist of fibers of protein called keratin. Collagen is the protein that strengthens your skin, blood vessels, bones and teeth. Muscles are held together by the protein fibers called myosin and actin. In fact, about one-fifth of your body weight is protein. Every chemical reaction that takes place in your body — that is a lot — is dependent on proteins. These important nutrients help us build new cells and repair damaged body tissue. Because your tissues are constantly being destroyed and rebuilt, and because unlike carbohydrates your body has no means to store protein, you must make sure you get enough of this important nutrient to keep all your vital processes functioning. During digestion, large molecules of protein are broken down into smaller, simpler units called amino acids. The body requires 22 amino acids in specific patterns to make human protein and thus do its necessary functions. Your body can produce all but nine of these amino acids. The nine that can not be produced are called essential amino acids because they must be supplied by your diet. In order for your body to properly use proteins, all of the essential amino acids must be present in your system. A food that contains all the essential amino acids is called a complete protein. Examples of foods high in protein include: meats, fish, lentils, and nuts, dairy products such as cheese or yogurt and beans.

Foods are Rich in Protein

Foods are rich in protein... meats (all sorts including fish and poultry), eggs, cheese, milk, legumes and nuts. Some of these foods have more protein in them than others, and some also have more fats in them than others. meat, a food from muscle, contains a lot of protein back when you learned that muscle is full of actin and myosin in order to contract. When we eat protein, we eat macromolecules.

Role of Protein

Proteins have a myriad of functions in our bodies, including as enzymes, receptors, hormones, membrane-proteins, cytoskeleton building blocks, and structural proteins. For example, our nails and hair are mainly made up of proteins manufactured by our skin. And many hormones that have to be continually made, like insulin, are proteins. Without proteins, we would structurally and biochemical fall apart!

Composition of Protein

The building blocks of proteins are amino acids, as you recently reviewed in Unit 23. When we eat protein, we have to break it down into its amino acids for absorption in the small intestines. After amino acids are absorbed, we can then use them to synthesize the proteins that our cells need. For example, when you eat eggs, the main protein you ingest is one called ovalbumin (similar to albumin); our bodies break that down into amino acids, and then we can make keratin or enzymes or fibrinogen, or whatever we need. We can totally recycle the ovalbumin amino acids into new proteins... It's kind of like being able to disassemble a desk in order to make a chair and footstool from the parts.

Storing Protein

The cells in our bodies are constantly making and breaking down proteins. There are normal anabolic and catabolic reactions to do this. In order to build a protein you must already have most of the amino acids... that is because there are some essential amino acids that we cannot make but that we have to ingest. There are 20 amino acids that we use to make proteins, and 8 of them (10 in children) are essential amino acids. When we breakdown proteins, much of the time we can just recycle the amino acids into new proteins that we are going to make.

However, when we breakdown proteins in order to make energy, like when we haven't eaten any carbohydrates in a while, the reaction (gluconeogenesis) plucks off the nitrogen portion of the amino acids from the proteins and dumps this portion as nitrogenous waste. This nitrogenous waste is cellular waste, and is removed from our bodies by the urinary system.

Requirement of Protein for Body

Your book describes needing approximately 0.4 grams of protein per pound of body weight. Let's assume that our class average body weight is 150 pounds (I am assuming that I skew us toward a heavier than normal amount!), then that means that we each have to take in 60 grams of protein per day. Converted into ounces, that means that we only have to each take in approximately 2 ounces of protein per day!

If we put that back together with our carbohydrate amount (approximately 9 oz) and the amount of lipid we should have in a day (no more than 30 per cent of total), if we eat 15 oz of food each day, 9 oz from carbohydrates, 2 oz from protein, and 4 oz of fat, we will have taken in all that we need. I guess the reason that I because the average weight to be so high is that I hardly ever eat less than one pound of food in a day!

In addition to our need for proteins, carbohydrates, nucleic acids, and lipids in our diets, we also need some other molecules. Some of these molecules are also organic molecules, and therefore contain carbon and hydrogen atoms within them. These additional organic molecules that we need are called vitamins. Other molecules that we need in our diets are not organic, and are called minerals.

Protein Need

After water, the biggest component in your body is protein. Over 98 per cent of the molecules in your body are replaced every year. So you need protein as a building block. If you don't get enough protein, or if you are eating poor quality protein, your body will not grow strong muscles, bones, blood, teeth, etc.

The eat right for your blood type diet's Peter D'Adamo recommends different ratios for each blood type. His rough guidelines are 20 per cent for A and AB, 34 per cent for B, and 45 per cent for O types. The metabolic diets don't specify protein requirements in grams, but Hunter-Gatherers need animal protein at every meal, whereas extreme Agriculturists thrive on a vegetarian diet.

Traditional nutritionists will probably recommend 10-15 per cent of calories. A lot of naturopathic nutritionists are concerned that the level of protein consumption is too high. I have seen recommendations ranging from 6 g/kg/day to 1 g/kg/day.

3

Carbohydrates

Starches and sugars are carbohydrates, the main source of the body's energy. Carbohydrates account for about half of the calorie intake for most Americans and up to four-fifths of the calories in diets of African and Asian peoples. Carbohydrate rich foods are also the main sources of protein for most of the world. Rice, wheat, corn, and potatoes are common rich sources of carbohydrates.

Sugars are not essential foods. They provide energy (calories) but no nutrients. For that reason sugar is called an "empty calorie" food. Occasional sweets are not harmful to a healthy, active person, but excessive sugar can lead to tooth decay when eaten between meals, especially in sticky snack foods that cling to the teeth. (See also carbohydrates)

Most of our energy comes from carbohydrates. Carbohydrates are chemical compounds of carbon, hydrogen and oxygen. They provide us with calories which can be converted into energy. There are two types of carbohydrates: simple, which are sugars, or complex, which are starches. It's a good idea to try to eat more complex carbohydrates because your body get longer sustained energy from these foods. Examples of complex carbohydrates include: potatoes, pasta, bread, rice, lentils, cereals and fruits and vegetables. Compare these to the simple carbohydrates such as cookies, candy bars and other sugar foods which provide a quick jolt of energy, but then leave your body craving more. These simple carbohydrates are known as "empty calories" because they lack vitamins, minerals, fiber or anything of value to your system.

Composition of Carbohydrates

Carbohydrates are polysaccharides and sugars. The most common and useful polysaccharides are starch (found only in plants) and glycogen (found mainly in muscle, or meat, and the liver). You see, when a plant has made (through photosynthesis) plenty of monosaccharide, it needs to store them for later use (like at night when it is dark outside). So the plant stores these monosaccharides (simple sugars) as starch. Meanwhile, in animals, we need the monosaccharides anywhere in our bodies where we need to make lots of ATP— and muscle is certainly a place for that! So, our muscles gather up the monosaccharides and store them as glycogen for later use. Therefore, when we look for food that is rich in polysaccharides, we typically look at foods derived from starchy plants and at meat.

Another polysaccharide that we eat is cellulose. It is the carbohydrate that makes up the cell walls of plant cells, and provides tough structure for the plants (since they lack bones). We have difficult time digesting cellulose, and, as mentioned in Unit 24, we rely on beneficial bacteria in our small intestines to get any of the monosaccharides out of cellulose. However, most of the cellulose we ingest still passes through our digestive system as unabsorbable material. Even though it is unabsorbed, it is useful in that it provides the fiber (a.k.a., roughage or bulk) in our diets that helps peristalsis of the alimentary canal to be effective.

Some disaccharides and monosaccharides in our diets. Common table sugar is a disaccharide. And anyone who has ever been around a kid after he/she has eaten a lot of sugar knows that the kid's digestive system was able to pick up a lot of sugars from that meal!

Role of Carbohydrate

Carbohydrates are used with oxygen to perform cellular respiration and produce ATP. Without carbohydrates we would run out of energy and our cells would die. Therefore, if we don't have enough available, we will make more from other molecules.

Micronutrients of Carbohydrate

Monosaccharides (or simple sugars) are the absorbable micronutrients of the carbohydrates. All monosaccharides have the same molecular formula of $C_6H_{12}O_6$. These atoms can be put together in a variety of ways, so there are multiple types of monosaccharides. The most important one is glucose, since it is vital for cellular respiration (even without oxygen it can be used to make ATP and build up lactic acid). There are other monosaccharides, like fructose and galactose, but these can be converted into glucose within liver cells in order to be more useful.

Storing Carbohydrates

Glycogensis. Literally, the making of glycogen. Glycogen is our storage polysaccharide for glucose, so, if we have a lot of glucose running around in our bodies, we convert it into glycogen using the chemical reactions called glycogen sis.

Glycogenolysis. Literally, the breakdown of glycogen. When glucose is in short supply, we breakdown any glycogen that we have (glycogen isn't typically for long-term storage).

Gluconeogenesis. When we do not have enough glucose and we have no more glycogen, we still need to make glucose available

Carbohydrate Need

It depends on how active we are. The more active, the more carbohydrates are needed. Your book says that an average person takes in 200-300 grams of carbohydrates daily—of that amount, somewhere around 150 grams is absolutely necessary if you are not going to break down proteins to make your energy. Converted into ounces, 200-300 g is the same as approximately 7-10 oz. This amount is only the amount of *usable* carbohydrates that we take in each day... it does not include the roughage in our diets.

Requirement of Carbohydrate

Protein, essential fats and micronutrients are primarily used as building materials. Carbohydrate is the only nutrient whose primary role is as fuel. To get lean, we want to burn up our supplies of excess fat, but to get consistently good performance, we need to give our bodies the right kind of fuel at the right time.

During exercise, we use ATP (adenosine troposphere) which our bodies can get more easily from muscle glycogen and blood glucose than from stored fat. Muscle glycogen comes from blood glucose, which comes from the carbohydrates that we eat.

Peter D'adamo (Eat Right For Your Blood Type) recommends different ratios for each blood type. His rough guidelines are 72 per cent for A, 60 per cent for AB, 56 per cent for B, and 38 per cent for O types. The metabolic diets range from minimal carbohydrates for extreme Hunter-Gatherers to high carbohydrates for extreme Agriculturists. Traditional nutritionists and naturopaths tend to favour high carbohydrates diets.

4

Fats

While too much fat is bad for your health, we do need some to survive. By cutting down on your fat intake you can reduce your chances of developing heart disease or cancer, not to mention staying in better physical shape and maintaining a healthy weight. There are three types of fat: saturated, monounsaturated and polyunsaturated. Saturated fats are the worst type because they raise the cholesterol level in your blood, which can lead to heart disease. The more saturated the fat is, the more solid it will appear at room temperature. This includes animal products such as butter, cheese, milk and meats. Monounsaturated fats are the types in nuts and fruit and polyunsaturated fats are found in oils. If you are trying to reduce the fat content in your diet, try broiling rather than frying your food, use skim milk rather than whole milk, use low-fat salad dressing or yogurt, and cut down on red meats.

Lipids are Fats

Remember, lipids are not made out of building blocks like carbohydrates, proteins, and nucleic acids. Instead, there are just different types of lipids. Here are the types of lipids that you have learned about:

1. Triglycerides (oils and lard)
2. Phospholipids (membrane lipids)
3. Steroids (cholesterol and hormones).

The main thing that these types of lipids have in

common is that they are all insoluble in water. Also, triglycerides and phospholipids both contain fatty acids and glycerol.

Role of Lipids

As far as quantity of a type of lipid, we mainly ingest triglycerides. We get them whenever we eat butter, oil, or animal fat. Of course, we also get phospholipids and steroids (mainly cholesterol) in our diets, just not as much as the triglycerides. A few phospholipids that we need are ones with fatty acids that we cannot make from scratch—therefore, we have to ingest certain fatty acids. The fatty acids that we have to ingest are called essential fatty acids (and we get them in our normal diets).

Triglycerides are mainly used for energy or energy reserves. You see, we can breakdown triglycerides and use the products of this breakdown for cellular respiration, or we can store triglycerides as fat. This requires a bit more of an explanation. After we eat triglycerides, our digestive system breaks them down into fatty acids and glycerol for absorption. The fatty acids are absorbed for the production of chylomicrons. Fatty acids enter the epithelial cells of the small intestine and are turned into chylomicrons with the help of the smooth endoplasmic reticulum. Once the chylomicrons are formed, they diffuse into the lacteal and eventually find their way back into the blood. Fatty acids can be drawn out of the chylomicrons into tissues that need them as the chylomicrons travel through the blood.

Fatty acids can be used in cellular respiration—they do not have to be turned into glucose first. Instead, the fatty acids are broken down into 2-carbon molecules that enter the cellular respiration events to make ATP. You see, glucose, a 6-carbon molecule, gets broken down into 3-carbon and then 2-carbon molecules as it goes through cellular respiration. Therefore, the 2-carbon molecules from fatty acids just join into the process where the 2-carbon molecules are normally used. Because they join in a little late in the process, they don't yield as much energy as glucose does, but they still generate some ATP.

Fatty acids can also be used to build storage triglycerides (fat for later use) and phospholipids for our membranes.

Cholesterol is important for manufacturing certain hormones, for helping to make up the lipid bilayer of cells, and for making bile salts.

Micronutrients of Lipid

There really isn't such a thing. Fatty acids and steroids are about as small as they get.

Storing Lipids

In the carbohydrate gave you names for the chemical reactions that occur to make or breakdown carbohydrates. Here, there are no analogous names that you need to know. But, I would like you to know that the liver orchestrates the breakdown and synthesis of lipids.

Need of Lipids

We don't need much lipid—only enough to get the essential fatty acids. Other than that, we can always make what we need. It is recommended that a person eat less than 30% of their daily calories from lipids

There are three main ways the body uses fats:

- *Structural*. Our bodies need fat as a building block. It is incorporated into cell membranes and other body structures, and used in fatty tissue.

- *Metabolic.* Affects hormones, including prostaglandins which affect metabolism.

- *As fuel.* It can be burned for energy. In fact, it is the body's preferred source of energy.

As well as that, fats are a valuable source of micronutrients, some of which can't be obtained from other foods.

So it is very important to eat enough fat, but also to make sure we eat the right kinds of fats. The wrong ones can have a profound effect on many body functions. There are two main debates about fat–how much you should eat, and which kinds you should eat. Let's look first at the different types of fat.

Types of Fat

There are several different ways of defining fats:

- Degree of saturation – saturated, monounsaturated and polyunsaturated. This is the main way that people differentiate fats and we'll go into that in more depth shortly.
- *Animal fats vs. vegetable oils.* This largely ties in with degree of saturation, with animal fats and tropical oils being mostly saturated, and vegetable oils being mostly unsaturated.
- *Chain length.* Short and medium chain fatty acids are found in butterfat and tropical oils, have anti-microbial and immune enhancing properties and are easily absorbed for energy, making them less likely to cause weight gain. This is why MCT (or Medium Chain Triglycerides) are often used in sports supplements. Unsaturated fats are generally made up of long or very long chain fatty acids.
- *Cist form vs. Trans form.* In nature, most fats occur in a "cist" form. In this form, they "fit" the fat receptors in your body, and can be utilized. Modern

processing methods (including heating, hydrogenation, bleaching and deodorizing) turn cist fats into trans fats, which no longer fit. Your body still tries to use them, but they don't do the job properly and disrupt your cellular metabolism, resulting in a variety of health hazards.

Saturated Fats

Saturated fats are straight chains of carbon and hydrogen that pack together easily so that they are relatively solid at room temperature. They are found predominantly in animal products and tropical oils.

Monounsaturated Fats

Monounsaturated fats have one double carbon bond, which means they are missing two hydrogen atoms. They are usually liquid at room temperature, but solidify when refrigerated. They are quite stable. They are mostly found in olives, nuts and avocados.

Polyunsaturated Fats

Polyunsaturated fatty acids come mostly from oils extracted from seeds. Their molecules have kinks in them at the point of the unsaturated double bonds. They do not pack together easily and therefore tend to be liquid at room temperature. These oils are extremely unstable and go rancid very easily.

5

Vitamins and Minerals

These nutrients don't supply your body with energy because they don't have calories. However, they are necessary because they help your body convert food into energy. Using our car analogy, vitamins and minerals are like spark plugs in a car, not the gas. The thirteen Vitamins A, C, D, E, K and the eight B vitamins (thiamine, riboflavin, niacin, B_6, pantothenic acid, biotin, folacin, and B_{12}) can be divided into two types: fat-soluble and water-soluble. You do not need to consume the fat-soluble vitamins everyday in order to maintain their proper levels because they are stored in your body fat and liver. But, the water-soluble vitamins, the B-complex vitamins and C, dissolve in the water in your system. So, these vitamins should be consumed everyday (with the exception of B_{12}, which your liver stores).

Vitamin A Promotes normal bone growth, healthy skin, hair and eyes, helps with night vision.

Vitamin C Strengthens blood vessels, helps the immune system, heals wounds and helps heal broken bones.

Vitamin D Helps absorb calcium for strong bones and teeth, your body produces this from sunlight.

Vitamin E Ensures that Vitamins A and C are not destroyed by oxygen and are properly used by your body. Helps form red blood cells.

Vitamin K	Called the clotting-factor vitamin, it enables your liver to produce a blood-clotting factor to control and prevent internal bleeding.
Vitamin B-Complex (8 different vitamins and minerals)	Breaks down carbohydrates and fat to energy, works to give you a healthy nervous system and healthy skin, helps you digest food and utilize minerals in foods you eat, important in the production of red blood cells, and works with proteins to build and repair tissues.
Thiamine	Helps keep your nervous system healthy, breaks down (Vit. B_1) carbohydrates into energy.
Riboflavin	Breaks down carbs, proteins and fats so your body can use (Vit. B_2) them for energy and repair.
Niacin	Works with riboflavin to convert proteins into energy. (Vit. B_3)
Calcium	Needed for healthy bone and teeth development, helps with muscle function, and helps blood to clot.
Iron	Ensures the body produces red blood cells—which transport oxygen. (Needed to produce hemoglobin–the red oxygen carrying pigment in blood.)
Folic acid	Needed to produce genetic material (DNA and RNA), needed during and before pregnancy to prevent birth defects.

Vitamin Classification

Fat Soluble Vitamins	***Water Soluble Vitamins***
Vitamin A	Vitamin B_1 (Thiamin)
Vitamin D	Vitamin B_2 (Riboflavin)
Vitamin E	Vitamin B_3 (Niacin)

Vitamin K

Vitamin B_5 (Pantothenic acid)
Vitamin B_6 (Pyridoxine)
Vitamin B_{12} (Cyanocobalamin)
Folic acid
Inositol
Choline
Vitamin C

Mineral Classification

Minerals	***Minerals***
Calcium	Copper
Magnesium	Manganese
Potassium	Chromium
Phosphorus	Selenium
Sodium	Iodine
Chloride	Molybelenum
Iron	Boron
Zinc	Fluoride
	Silica
	Cobalt
	Nickel

Calcium

Calcium is needed for strong, healthy bones and teeth. Women, especially post-menopausal, are in danger of developing osteoporosis if their intake is not sufficient. It is also necessary for correct muscle and nerve action, it helps maintain blood acidity and assists in blood clotting, and maintains healthy skin.

Signs of Calcium Deficiency

Shrinkage of skeleton, osteoporosis, muscle cramps, tingling or trembling, eye cataracts, slow blood clotting, irregular heart beat, irritability, insomnia and mental disorders.

Copper

Copper is a trace mineral found in all body tissues. It helps the body absorb iron, helps regulate and stimulate the brain, helps protect and support the nervous and glandular systems, assists in forming muscle and bone, and assists in the pigmentation of hair and skin.

Signs of Copper Deficiency

Too little copper can cause fatigue, weak blood cells, impaired respiration, skin sores, and lack of hair and skin pigmentation. Copper deficiencies are fairly rare, but can be caused by mega doses of zinc or Vitamin C.

Types of Vitamins and Minerals

There are many types of vitamins. Some vitamins are water soluble, while others are not. Some are needed to make other molecules in our cells (like Vitamin A is needed to make the rhodopsin pigment in our retinas), others are needed to promote absorption of materials in our digestive system (like Vitamin D facilitates calcium absorption), others can be used as coenzymes (interacting with enzymes to increase their functionality), and there are even more functions that we do not need to worry about in this course. Some our bodies can synthesize (like Vitamin D if exposed to sunlight), and others we can only obtain by ingesting them (like Vitamin C). If we must ingest them in our diets, as is more typical with vitamins, they are called essential vitamins.

Minerals tend to be those elements that we need in small amounts, and we obtain them as atoms rather than in large molecules. For example, you know that iron atoms are needed in every hemoglobin molecule for it to work properly. Well, we lose some iron atoms every day and need to replace them in order to keep our hemoglobin working well. Therefore, we must get iron in our diets. That is pretty simple if you eat meat, because meat contains some blood within it, and that blood has hemoglobin with iron in it. It is also pretty easy because if the meat you eat is liver, where iron is stored for recycling, you'll get tons of it. But, you can see, you have to eat the right foods to get the needed minerals. Or, you can take a vitamin and mineral pill to get them. Any way you go about it, though, you will need to ingest minerals.

6

Energy

To understand this, you will need to remember a basic principle (of thermodynamics) that you have learned somewhere before in your educational career: *energy cannot be created or destroyed, but it can be converted from one form into another.* Energy has many forms... one form is chemical energy, which is the type stored within chemical bonds in molecules like glucose and ATP. Another type of energy is heat. You have already seen, back in the muscle chapter, that when we use lots of ATP in our muscles, like during a long workout, some of the energy from the ATP is lost as heat, and so our muscles heat up. That is an example of energy changing forms. Therefore, energy can be measured as chemical energy or heat energy, or even other types of energy. But the easiest measurement to make is in terms of heat—all you need is a thermometer! So, energy is typically measured in heat units called *calories.*

Calories relate back to the temperature you would measure with a thermometer in the following way. If 1000 calories of heat are released in water, the temperature of the water would increase by 1°C. Water is specified, because different materials accept heat (conduct heat) differently. Nutritionists need to be able to talk about a lot of calories, so it is more useful for nutritionists to talk about *kilocalories* (which are also called *calories* with a capital "C" or "large calories"). A kilocalorie, abbreviated *kcal* or just *cal,* is the amount of heat required to raise the temperature of water 1°C, and is equal to 1000 calories.

One can relate the amount of each organic molecule consumed back to its caloric equivalence. So, 1 gram of either carbohydrates or proteins yields 4.1 calories of energy. And 1 gram of fats ingested yields 9.5 calories (more than double the amount carbohydrates and proteins yield).

Energy Needs

The amount of energy that we need can be described by our rate of energy consumption. Let's consider our rate of energy consumption at times when we are resting. This rate is called the *basal metabolic rate,* or *BMR.* If you think about it, the amount of energy that we consume should be proportional to the amount of energy that we make. And the amount of energy that we make stems from our rate of cellular respiration. The rate of cellular respiration is mainly dependent on our aerobic respiration, which requires oxygen (and glucose or its breakdown products) to occur. Therefore, BMR is proportional to the rate of our oxygen consumption. So, one's BMR can be evaluated somewhat by one's rate and volume of breathing at rest.

On average, a person's BMR is one kcal/hr for each kilogram (kg) of body weight. Since 1 kg = 2.7 lb, a person with a body weight of 150 lb can also be described as having a body weight of 55.6 kg. This person would then use at least 55.6 kcal every hour of every day. Over 24 hours this person would use 1362 kcal. This number of 1362 kcal would require that our average person be lying down and not doing anything for all 24 hours. Even just sitting up would increase energy consumption. You how many more calories (NOT kcal, even though they capitalize it) per hour a person would consume by various activities. For example, just walking around at a slow, meandering pace consumes 200 extra calories per hour, or (200 cal * 12 hr =) 2400 cal, or 2.4 kcal extra if you walk around for half the day.

Your energy needs are equal to the amount of energy you will be using in the day. You need to consume a little more than just your energy needs in order to replenish your essential-nutrients-stock. However, to maintain your weight, you should not eat much more than what you will use in a day. For example, if you eat an additional 3500 calories in a day, over the amount you will use, you will gain one pound.

7

Meal Planning for an Individual

Introduction

The members of a family often have different food requirements. Their preferences as regards the foods also very. Some members have sweets while others prefer family tasty savour dishes. Hence you may need large member of dishes a single meal to meet family food requirements. This situation is neither practical nor economical. Careful meal planning caters to most of the family needs, likes and dislikes.

What is Meal Planning

It is a technique of providing the family with meals that will meet their nutritional requirement. Meal planning is an Art as well a science. The meals served is an attractive way stimulate one's desire to eat. An individual salivates easily at the prefect of good taste. The digestive juices thus secreted go a long way in helping the body desire maximum food value. It is often called science because the knowledge of scientific principles of nutrition guide the home maker is making ins from the variety of foods available for optimum nutrition to all members of the family.

Hence, meal planning can be defined as the "implementation of the principles of nutrition in one's daily diet is an appetizing way".

The daily requirements of various foods are

distributed over the day in different meals. In an urban family the meals are breakfast, lunch, evening tea and dinner. This meal pattern is not rigid, hence, if can be varied to suit the and individual and family needs.

Importance of Meal Planning

All family members do not have the same nutrition requirements. Children eat less food than the adults. Grandfather may not be eating sweets because he is diabetic. Hence you ever seen a labourer eating his meal? He eats much more than your father. Hence meal planning is a very carefully drawn out plan of serving adequate meals to all the members of the family. The important factors of meal planning are as follows:

(a) Nutritional needs.
(b) Personal likes and dislikes.
(c) Serving attractive meals.
(d) Planning nutritional meals within the family budget.
(e) Good food combination.
(f) Using left over foods.
(g) Serving time, energy and fuel.

(a) Nutritional Needs: The protein requirement are high among growing children and hence they should be given sufficient amount of proteins of high biological value, e.g. milk, egg, and soybean etc. The protein requirements also increase during pregnancy and lactation. After operations and individual should have high protein diet to promote to promote recovery. The calories requirements are high among active adolescent boys and girls. Athletes and labourers do strenuous exercise and work, thus require more of energy giving foods.

(b) Personal Likes and Dislike: The meals planned for any individual should take into account his/ her preferences. Children often dislike drinking milk which is an important source of most nutrients. Hence the milk can be given to them in the form of *Kheer*, custard or curd and the ice-cream that will be acceptable to the as far as possible there should be no compromise of nutritional needs on account of personal preferences.

(c) Serving Attractive Meals: I well planned meal should be appealing to the eyes. When you see an attractively served meat it creates an intense desire to eat it. It is rightly said that one eats with eyes finest. On the other hand what will your reaction be. If you are asked to take the sloppily served meal? Public eating places lay a lot of emphasis an garnishing and serving dishes to the customers. An intelligent mother and home maker will put in her best to provide attractive meals to her family. Her efforts will ensure good health for the family.

(d) Planning Nutritional Meals within the Family Budget: Food is expensive and hence a large chunk of one's income goes into the kitchen in order to provide balanced diet for all members of the family:

(i) Milk, meat and meat products provide A grade protein and these are expensive well informed housewife can use attractive foods to effect economy. Soyabeans and soyabean preparations can at times replace meat, chicken, etc. to cut down the food cast.

(ii) Seasonal foods are often cheaper than the off-seasons and convenience foods. Seasonal foods besides being tastier can affect economy. Seasonal foods are nutritionally superior to off-season and convenient foods.

(iii) You get iron from green leafy vegetables. It is a common practice to discard radish leaves and eat the white root eating. Cook the green radish leaves, and you have a dish providing you iron at no additional cost.

(iv) Lemons, orange and lime are expensive sources of Vitamin E. Amla, guava, and fresh salads provide all Vitamin C. You need, but at relationally less cost. Experience and awareness as regards different foods will equip you to serve low cost but nourishing and healthy meals for your family.

(e) Good Food Combination: It enables one to plan balanced meals for the family. Rice is deficient in lysine and pulses are deficient in methionine. The protein content thus improves if nice, and deal are taken together. *Khichri*, idle, dosa are some examples of good food combinations.

Deal are food sources of protein but when cooked in combination with green leafy vegetable improve considerably in iron content. Potatoes provide carbohydrates of combine well with a variety foods for making nutrition dishes. Can you name some of these dishes? Yes *potato pea curry, potato methi, potato palak bhujia, potato pakodas and potato sprouted moong daal chaat* etc.

(f) Using Left Over Foods: It is important to incorporate left over foods to make a new dish. This way the monotony of eating the same foods, and the wastage can be avoided. Supposing your have left over deal, what can you make with it? Knead daal with atta, add coriander leaves, green chilies and chopped onion and make parathas with it. It sounds pretty in pressing to pack with paratha in your tiffin box. Boiled rice can be used to *kheer*, and lemon rice. Hence, the meal planning ensures prefer use of left over foods together with money saving.

(g) Saving Time, Energy and Fuel: Planning of meals avoids unnecessary trips to the market to procure required food items. Planning of meals ensures organized shopping, thus saving on both time and energy. Items required in large amounts also cast less when purchased in bulk.

It is desirable to use appropriate and simple methods of cooking to same fuel. You have studied the different methods of cooking in your previous class. This knowledge will enable you to cook foods for maximum nutritive value cook foods having simple recipes. Avoid lengthy cooking to conserve fuel. Make maximum use of pressure cooker. Use pressure cooker containers to cook more than one food at a time. It conserve a lot of fuel which is a lime resources.

Advantages of Meal Planning

The advantages of meal planning can be summed up as follows:

- It fulfils the nutritional needs of all family members.
- Attractive meals can be served with prior meal planning.
- Planning keeps individual likes and dislikes in mind and alternative nutritional meal can be made without compromising on nutrients.
- Proper meal planning saves money, time, energy and fuel.
- Different foods can be combined for increment of nutrient intake.
- Left over foods can be effectively used.

Factors Affecting Meal Planning

No two individual on families have exactly the same nutritional needs. Hence their diets differ in order to meet their physical, social and psychological needs. There are a member of factors which play an important role in meal planning.

(1) Adequacy of Food: A good mean is one which will not only provide adequate accounts of fats, Calories, and proteins but also minerals and vitamins essential for the physical well being of each members of the family. Therefore, the age, sex, occupation, physiological condition and member of family members must be kept in mind. Hence for meals may very widely but an attempt must be made to provide a diet that will not lead to protein deficiency accompanied by a deficiency of iron. Sometimes deficiency of milk leads to a diet which is low in calcium. The one on more foods from each of the different groups discussed will prevent most imbalances in diets.

(2) Meal Patterns must Fulfill the Family Needs: While planning needs, one should candidate the needs and requirements of each individual member of the family. In a family there maybe a child, a man, adolescent boy and girl etc. Housewife who plans the meals has to see to their different nutritional requirements.

(3) Meal Planning should Save Time and Energy and Result in Easy to Cook Meals: This point is particularly important for the families of low income groups or where the housewife is also working. If the meal consist of too many dishes and each takes a lot of time to prefer, then the housewife will spend for too meal time in the kitchen and become frustrated as other household chores remain complete.

(4) Individual Likes and Dislikes: Some people make personal likes and dislikes the only basis for the member on exclusion of certain foods in their meals – the failure to include milk is a common practice. It is always better to change the form of the food rather than to completely unit. For example, milk can be given in the form of curd, cheese, custard or another sweet dish, soyabeans in the forms of soya for *chapattis* mixed with wheat flour.

(5) Suitable Combination: Food in suitable ways, variety in meals can be obtained and variety in meals means acceptability, thus ensuring better nutrition. This can be introduced by changes in colour, shape, texture, flavours and methods of preparation. Attractive combination, texture varieties, Flavours and methods of cooking play important role in it.

(6) Food should Provide Satisfy Value: Food rich in protein and fasts have a higher satisfy value compared to carbohydrates. While planning consider the interval between the two meals and accordingly include foods. If the interval is longer, give foods rich in proteins and fats. If the interval is short, then give carbohydrates foods.

(7) Availability of Foods: The dietary habit depended mainly upon the foods produced a particular area or community, but today with improved methods of food preservation and distribution, even the mast perishable foods are available over large areas. The wide variation in dietary patterns throughout the world depends largely upon the available food supply.

(8) Economic Considerations: The budget of a family of moderate means cannot provide luxury foods but it can definitely offer variety and choice. Food budgets of low income groups restrict the choices still function and it may become necessary to depend largely on cereals foods. The problem faced then is the supplementation of these cereals with foods necessary for a balanced diet. Although it becomes difficult to plan, it is nevertheless possible. When the cost per day is low, it is very important to have a good knowledge of less expensive foods which have high nutritive value. Such recipes and foods should be included in meal preparation, e.g., *paustik roti*, seasonal vegetables, butter, milk, pickle or *chutney*.

(9) Seasonal Foods: Today the seasons play a less important role in meal planning then in former times because fresh frozen foods are available throughout the year. Still foods included in the diet plans should be season because they are cheap and available in food quality and are within the reach within the reach of all people.

(10) Religion, Traditions and Customs: This is an important factor and food habits must be kept in mind while planning meals because they differ form religion to religion. Muslims can not eat pork, where as Hindus cannot eat beef. Rice is considered as an auspicious dish at festivals and marriage. Widows are generally not served fish in Bengal. Customs and traditions differ from community to community and hence should be kept in view while planning meals for a family.

Occupations and Calorie Requirements

The approximate member of calories required per hour to perform different activities. These figures include the basal calories need.

Types of Activity	*Calorie/Hour*
(a) Sedentary activities Reading, writing, eating, watching TV, sewing, playing card, office sitting work	80-100
(b) Cooking food, dusting, hand washing, articles washing, ironing, walking personal care, typing, office work	110-160
(c) Moderate activities: making bed, moping, sweeping light gardening, walking fast, setting office work	170-240
(d) Vigorous activities:	250-350

heavy scrubbing and waxing, hand washing, cloth washing, hanging out clothes, stripping beds, other heavy work, golfing	
(e) Strenuous activities: swimming, playing, running, skipping, cycling, dancing	350 and more

Flexibility in Meal Planning

It is very important to allow a certain amount of flexibility while planning a meal for your family. You have planned to serve mutton stew to your family and just then your vegetation grandmother arrives. What will you do? Cook special food separately for your grandmother on make vegetable stew instead of the mutton stew. However the later option is better for the entire family can enjoy the same meal with the visiting grandmother.

You had planned a rich, elaborate menu for the entire family. This food plan should be flexible in case of some family member falls sick. There should be flexibility in interchanging lunch and dinner meals on say Monday meals to Tuesday meal etc.

Guidelines for Good Eating Habits

(a) Maintain regular eating routine.
(b) Eat a whole lot of natural foods.
(c) Eat just right amounts foods, neither more nor less.
(d) Consume seasonal foods.
(e) Avoid excessive consumption of salt, spices, fats, sugars and sweets.
(f) Eat carbohydrates that supply plenty of fiber.

(g) Eat variety as it ensures supply of all essential nutrients.
(h) Maintain desirable height and health.

Meal Planning for an Individual

Planning meal for an individual in a lot easier than planning the same for a family. Do you know why? Yes, you only have to take into consideration the requirements, likes and dislikes of only an individual.

Before you set out for planning meals refresh your knowledge about balanced diet and recommended dietary allowances (RDA). Given below is a sample menu for an adult women made for the recommended food allowances.

A Day's Sample Menu for an Adult Women

Name / Age		*Sudha / 30 years*
Structure	—	Medium
Activity	—	Moderate
Habit	—	Vegetarian
Food Allowances		
Cereals	—	350 gm
Pulses	—	70 gm
Green leaf vegetable	—	125 gm
Other vegetable	—	75 gm
Roots and tubers	—	75 gm
Fruits	—	30 gm
Milk	—	200 ml
Fat and oil	—	35 gm
Sugar and jaggery	—	30 gm
Recommended Dietary Allowances		
Calories	—	2225
Proteins	—	50 gm

Calcium	—	400 mg
Iron	—	30 mg
Vitamin A	—	2400 mg

Meal	*Menu*	*Nutrient*	*Provide*
BT	Tea	1 Cup	Carb.-Sugar
BF	Paustik roti/		
	Parathas	-2	Protein carb.
	And	½K	Protein
Lunch	Chapatti	3	Carb.
	Moong daal	1 K	Protein
	Carrot and methi veg.	½K	Vitamin A and I
	Papad	1	Protein
	Green chutney	1-2 Tsp.	Iron and Vitamin-C
	Radish and tomato	½Plate	Vitamin-C, Vitamin-A
Ev. Tea	Suji upma	1 K	Carb.
	Tea/Coffee	1 Cup	Carb-sugar
Dinner	Steamed rice	1 Plate	Card
	Rajmah curry	1 ½K	Protein
	Chapatti	1-2	Carb
	Aloo-brinjal veg.	1 K	Carb-roughages
	Banana-Custard	1 K	Carb, protein and calcium

Note: You can plan meals for different family members following the pattern just studied.

8

Food Preservation

Unless food is preserved in some manner, it begins to spoil soon after it is harvested or slaughtered. The main methods of food preservation that will keep food safe are canning, freezing and drying. Preserving food at home means having:

- An abundant supply of a variety of foods when the fresh products aren't readily available;
- Specialities such as strawberry-fig preserves or green tomato relish that can't always be purchased;
- The satisfaction of actually preserving foods yourself.

However, preserving food at home may not save you money, depending on the cost of buying or raising the food and the equipment, energy and time needed.

Canning

Canning is the process in which foods are placed in jars or cans and heated to a temperature that destroys microorganisms and inactivates enzymes. This heating and later cooling forms a vacuum seal. The vacuum seal prevents other microorganisms from recontaminations the food within the jar or can. High-acid foods such as fruits and tomatoes can be processed or "canned" in boiling water, while low-acid vegetables and meats must be processed in a pressure canner at 240°F (10 pounds pressure at sea level).

Pickling: It is another form of canning. Pickled products have an increased acidity that makes it difficult for most bacteria to grow. Pickled products are also heated in jars at boiling temperatures to destroy any other microorganisms present and form a vacuum in the jar.

Jams and Jellies: Have a very high sugar content. The sugar binds with the liquid present making it difficult for microorganisms to grow. To prevent surface contamination after the product is made and thus possible yeast or mold growth, jams and jellies are either canned, frozen or refrigerated.

Freezing

Freezing reduces the temperature of the food so that microorganisms cannot grow, yet some may still live. Enzyme activity is slowed down but not stopped during freezing.

Enzymes in Vegetables: These must be inactivated by blanching in order to prevent loss of colour, flavour and nutrients. The vegetable is exposed to boiling water or steam for a specified time and then quickly cooled in ice water to prevent cooking. Blanching also helps to destroy microorganisms on the surface of the vegetable.

Enzymes in Fruits: These can cause browning and loss of Vitamin C, and are controlled by the addition of ascorbic acid.

Drying

Drying removes most of the moisture from foods. Thus microorganisms cannot grow and enzyme action is slowed down. Dried foods should be stored in airtight containers to prevent moisture from dehydrating the products and allowing microbial growth.

Unsafe Canning Methods

Open-kettle Method: This outdated method of canning is now considered unsafe. In this method, foods were heated in a kettle, then poured into jars and a lid was placed on the jar. No processing was done. With this method there was often spoilage because bacteria, yeast and molds that contaminated the foods when the jars were filled were not killed by further processing. The growth of these microorganisms, in addition to spoiling the food, often caused any lids that did seal to later come unsealed

Steam Canning: This is a newer method of canning that is not considered safe at this time. The jars are heated by steam. However, safe processing times have not been developed and steam canners are NOT recommended for either high- or low-acid foods. Low-acid foods canned in these canners are potentially deadly because of possible botulism contamination. Also, both low- and high-acid foods are often very under processed and therefore could spoil.

Other Unsafe Methods: Canning food in the microwave oven, electric ovens, slow cookers or crock pots can be extremely dangerous, especially with low-acid foods, and is not recommended. So-called canning powders are useless as preservatives and do not replace the need for proper heat processing.

Adjustments for Altitudes

As altitude increases, water boils at lower temperatures. Because the lower temperatures are less effective for killing bacteria, the processing time must be increased for boiling water bath canning. For pressure canning, the pressure is increased.

The directions for canning foods are usually for an altitude of 0 to 1000 feet. If you are canning at an altitude over 1000 feet, check for altitude adjustments needed for canning each type of food.

On Guard Against Spoilage

Don't taste or use food that shows any kind of

spoilage! Look closely at all jars before opening them. A bulging lid or leaking jar is a sign of spoilage. When you open the jar, look for other signs, such as spurting liquid and off-odours or mold.

Spoiled canned foods should be discarded in a place where they will not be eaten by humans or pets. Spoiled meats, seafood and low-acid vegetables, should be detoxified to destroy any poisons that might be present before they are discarded.

To detoxify canned low-acid foods that have been spoiled, carefully remove the lid from the jar. Place the jar(s) of food and the lids in a saucepot. (No need to remove the food from the jar — removing it could contaminate other items.) Add enough hot water to cover the jar(s). Boil for 30 minutes and then cool. Drain water and dispose of food and lids. The jars may be reused.

Improperly canned low-acid foods can contain without showing signs of spoilage. Low-acid foods are considered improperly canned and not safe if any of the following are true:

- the food was not processed in a pressure canner.
- the gauge of the canner was inaccurate.
- up-to-date researched processing times and pressures were not used for the size of the jar, style of pack and kind of food being processed.
- ingredients were added that were not in an approved recipe.
- proportions of ingredients were changed from the original approved recipe.
- the processing time and pressure were not correct for the altitude at which the food was canned.

Because improperly canned low-acid foods can contain botulinum toxin without showing signs of spoilage, they should also be detoxified and then discarded.

Surfaces that come in contact with spoiled or questionable food should be cleaned with a solution of 1 part chlorine bleach to 5 parts water. Wet the surface with this solution and let stand 5 minutes before rinsing.

Preserving Food for Special Diets

It is possible to preserve food at home for people who are watching their salt or sugar intakes. Simply use methods that don't require sugar or salt for their preservative properties.

If preserving food for someone trying to cut sugar consumption, the food may be dried, or fruits may be canned or frozen in water or juice instead of a sugar syrup. The sugar specified in canning and freezing is only needed for its effects on flavour and texture. There are also many pickle recipes that call for little or no sugar. Sugar is the major means by which most jams, jellies and preserves are safely preserved. These products are not suitable for a person on a low-sugar diet. However, there are special low-methoxyl pectins and recipes designed to make jams and jellies with no added sugar.

It is also possible to preserve food at home for people who are watching their salt intake. The salt used in canning, freezing or drying foods is used only for its flavour or colour protection quality. Pickling, especially when fermentation is involved, usually requires salt for preservative effect. Read the recipe. If it calls for a large quantity of salt, this can not be eliminated or replaced with a salt substitute. However, if the recipe calls for a large amount of vinegar and only a teaspoon or two of salt for flavour (not soaking), the salt can be left out.

9

Food Groups

Basic Food Groups

A well-balanced diet offers you many mouth-watering food choices. With this helpful guide, you'll learn about AHA-recommended servings and sizes for each food group or specialized category. You'll also see how easy and fun it is to combine a wide variety of foods to create a well-balanced diet.

Each of the basic food groups supplies a different combination of nutrients, vitamins and minerals. Let caloric needs and a healthy appetite be your guide. But remember, variety is the key to good nutrition.

Bread, Cereal, Rice and Pasta

Grain products like bread, cereal, rice, and pasta are good for you. They are important sources of vitamins and minerals. Breads, cereals, rice, and pasta are also good sources of carbohydrates like starch and fiber.

Many people think that starchy foods like breads, rice and pasta are fattening. They are not. But when you add fats like margarine, oil, mayonnaise, cheese sauce or gravy to them, you add many extra calories. Whole-grain foods have more fiber than white grain foods. There are many kinds of whole-grain foods, such as oatmeal, brown rice, grits, corn tortillas and whole wheat bread. You may want to try a whole grain bread instead of white bread. Use brown rice instead of white rice or mix them together the next time you have rice.

Some breads and cereals have lots of fat and sugar added when they are manufactured. Croissants, danish, doughnuts, cake and some muffins have more fat and calories than servings of plain breads and cereals. If you enjoy sweet breads and cereals, you don't have to give them up. Try eating these foods less often or in small amounts. When you shop, read the food labels and look for breads, cereals, rice and pasta mixes that have less fat and sugar in them. You can also cut down on fat when you make rice or pasta dishes. Try using less oil, butter, or margarine than the recipe says. Sometimes you can cut the fat in half without changing the way the food tastes or looks.

Fats, Oils and Sweets

Fats, oils and sweets give us calories. Fats and oils like salad dressings, mayonnaise, butter, margarine and lard tend to be high in calories because of the fat they contain. Sweets like candy, soft drinks, syrups, jams, and jellies are made mostly of sugars. Most of these foods do not contain many vitamins or minerals. So they are called "empty calorie" foods.

Fats, oils and sweets are not bad foods. When we eat them along with foods like grains, fruits, vegetables, milk and meat products they are part of a healthy diet. Eating too many fats, oils or sweets can be a problem when we eat them instead of foods and nutrients we get in the other food groups.

Fats, oils and sweets add flavour and variety to our diets. We don't have to give them up. We can use less of them to help us stay fit and healthy. We can spread a smaller amount of butter, margarine or jelly on toast or muffins. We can use less fat and oil in cooking. When we cook we can cut down of some of the fats and sugars by reducing the amounts of these ingredients in the recipes we make.

Fruits

Fruits are important sources of vitamins and carbohydrates like fiber and sugar. They are low in calories and naturally sweet. Fruits and their juices are good sources of water, too.

Different fruits contain different vitamins, so it is important to eat a variety of fruits. Mangoes, papayas, melons and citrus fruits, like oranges and grapefruit, are high in Vitamin C. Cantaloupe, apricots, peaches, and nectarines are sources of Vitamin A.

Whole fruits like apples and grapes contain more fiber than fruit juices and sauces, like applesauce and grape juice. Dried fruits like figs, prunes and raisins are good sources of fiber, too. Canned fruits packed in syrup have a lot of added sugar. They are higher in calories than fresh fruits. When you shop for canned fruits, look for fruit that is packed in juice instead of syrup.

Meat, Poultry, Fish, Dry Beans, Eggs and Nuts

Meat, poultry, fish, dry beans, eggs, and nuts are important sources of protein, iron, zinc, and B vitamins. This group includes plant foods and animal foods.

Some meats and meat products are high in fat. There are many ways to reduce the fat you get from these meats. You can choose leaner cuts like chuck, bottom round or top round of beef, pork loin or lamb shank. You can trim fat from meat before cooking and eating. You can take the skin off chicken. Many processed meats like hot dogs, sausage, pepperoni, bacon, ham and luncheon meats are high in fat and sodium. If you enjoy eating these meats, try having them less often and when you do, try eating them in smaller amounts.

Because eggs are a good source of iron and protein, they are counted as a meat serving. Most of the fat in eggs is found in the yolk. When you use the egg whites, you can cut the fat and keep the protein and vitamins you need.

Plant foods like lentils, black-eyed peas, chick peas and other dried beans and peas are inexpensive sources of protein. Unlike meats, beans are low in fat and high in fiber. Nuts and nut butters like peanuts and peanut butter are good sources of protein and iron; but they are higher in fat than other plant foods.

You can get the nutrients you need from this group without a lot of fat and without costing a lot. Many lean meats like beef chuck are also lower in cost. If you buy ground beef that is 70 per cent fat because it is less expensive, you can still reduce the fat. Try draining the meat after you cook it or add other ingredients. Mix small amounts of meat with pasta, beans and rice to stretch your food dollar. You will get the same nutrients but it will cost you less.

Milk, Yogurt and Cheese

Milk and foods made from milk are the best sources of the mineral calcium. They also provide us with Vitamin A, protein and phosphorus. Fortified milk has Vitamin D added to it.

The foods in this group are important because all of the nutrients work together to keep our bones strong and healthy. It may be difficult to get enough calcium unless we include these foods in our diets. We can make sure we get the milk and calcium we need by making puddings and soups with milk.

Some milk products like ice-cream, cheese, whole milk and foods made from whole milk are high in fat. We can choose low-fat or skim milk products, like low-fat yogurt, skim milk and low-fat cheeses to keep the fat in our diets down.

Some people who have problems digesting milk products because of lactose (sugar) in milk. Today there are many lactose-free products to try.

Vegetables

Vegetables are a source of important vitamins, minerals and carbohydrates. Because vegetables differ in the vitamins and minerals they contain, it is important to eat a variety of vegetables. Cabbages, plantains, peppers and leafy green vegetables like poke greens and kale are rich sources of Vitamin C. Deep orange and dark green vegetables are high in Vitamin A. Broccoli, spinach, collards and kale are dark green vegetables that contain calcium and iron. Cabbage family vegetables like broccoli, cauliflower, turnips and rutabagas help prevent certain cancers.

Fresh vegetables are naturally low in fat, calories and sodium. Extra fat and calories can come from cooking or other types of processing. If you add fat, oil, margarine or lard when you cook vegetables, you also add fat and calories. If you buy frozen vegetables with special sauces, you may also be adding fat and calories. You can buy frozen vegetables without special sauces and get the same nutrients as fresh vegetables. Some canned vegetables have added salt. While the salt adds flavour, it also adds extra sodium to your diet. When you shop for canned vegetables, look for vegetables with no salt added.

Food Pyramid

The food guide pyramid has been rebuilt! The biggest change is that the food groups are no longer horizontal blocks of the pyramid. Now, a rainbow of coloured, vertical stripes represent the five food groups, as well as fats and oils. Here's what the colors stand for:

Orange	-	Grains
Green	-	Vegetables
Red	-	Fruits
Blue	-	Milk and dairy products
Purple	-	Meat, beans, fish and nuts
Yellow	-	Oils

Daily Requirements of Food Groups

Everyone wants to know how much they should eat to stay healthy. It's a tricky question, though. It depends on your age, whether you're a girl or a boy, and how active you are. Kids who are more active burn more calories so they need more calories. But we can give you some estimates for how much you need of each food group.

Grains

Grains are measured out in ounce equivalents. What the heck are they? Ounce equivalents are just another way of showing a serving size.

Here are ounce equivalents for common grain foods. An ounce equivalent equals:

1 piece of bread
1/2 cup of cooked cereal, like oatmeal
1/2 cup of rice or pasta
1 cup of cold cereal

4- to 8-year-old need 4 to 5 ounce equivalents each day.

9- to 13-year-old girls need 5 ounce equivalents each day.

9- to 13-year-old boys need 6 ounce equivalents each day.

And one last thing about grains: Try to eat a lot of whole grains, such as 100% wheat bread, brown rice, and oatmeal.

Vegetables

Of course, you need your vegetables, especially those dark green and orange ones. But how much is enough? Vegetable servings are measured in cups.

4- to 8-year-olds need 1-1/2 cups of veggies each day.
9- to 13-year-old girls need 2 cups of veggies each day.
9- to 13-year-old boys need 2-1/2 cups of veggies each day.

Fruits

Sweet, juicy fruit is definitely part of a healthy diet. Here's how much you need:

4- to 8-year-old need 1 cup to 1-1/2 cups of fruit each day.
9- to 13-year-old girls need 1 1/2 cups of fruit each day.
9- to 13-year-old boys need 1-1/2 cups of fruit each day.

Milk and Other Calcium-Rich Foods

Calcium builds strong bones to last a lifetime, so you need these foods in your diet.

4 to 8-year-olds need 1 cup to 2 cups of milk (or another calcium-rich food) each day.
9 to 13-year-old girls need 3 cups of milk (or another calcium-rich food) each day.
9 to 13-year-old boys need 3 cups of milk (or another calcium-rich food) each day.

If you want something other than milk, you can substitute yogurt, cheese, or calcium-fortified orange juice–just to name a few.

Meats, Beans, Fish and Nuts

These foods contain iron and lots of other important nutrients. Like grains, these foods are measured in ounce equivalents.

An ounce equivalent of this group would be:

1 ounce of meat, poultry, or fish
1/4 cup cooked dry beans
1 egg
1 tablespoon of peanut butter
A small handful of nuts or seeds
4 to 8-year-olds need 3 to 4 ounce equivalents each day.
9 to 13-year-old girls need 5 ounce equivalents each day .
9 to 13-year-old boys need 5 ounce equivalents each day.

Whoa! That's a lot to swallow. The good news is that your mom, dad, and the other grownups in your life will help you eat what you need to stay healthy. There's more good news–you don't have to become a perfect eater overnight. Just remember those stairs climbing up the side of the new pyramid and take it one step at a time.

10

Food Adulteration

Introduction

A variety of food and other items are purchased in all homes. A lot of one's hard earned money is spent on food alone. Have you cooked at the wheat that has been procured for your family?

Is it Clean?

Is the wheat mixed with similar cooking mud balls and some things?
Are all the grains healthy or some shrunken grains are also present in the wheat purchased?

Is the Wheat Worm-Infested?

You must be knowledgeable enough to distinguish between good quality and inferior quality foods. Make that you are not being cheated. It will also ensure that you get your money's worth.

After reading this chapter you will be able to:
- Define and explain the meaning of adulteration.
- Differentiate between adulterant and adulteration.
- Enumerate factors under which the food is considered adultered according to the Prevention of Food adulteration Act (PFA).
- Enlist some of the adulterate present in commonly used foods.
- Enumerate hazards due to commonly present adulterate.

- Discuss steps taken for protection against adulteration.
- Describe simple tests of defection of the adulterant present in the food.
- Enumerate the measures to safeguard against food adulteration.
- Appreciate that the standard marks safeguard the consumer against food adulteration.

Definition and Meaning of Adulteration

The food is considered adultered in the following instances:

(a) Addition of cheap and inferior substances lesser the quality of foods purchased. For example—Water in milk, vanaspati in pure ghee.

(b) Removal of valuable component also lowers and deteriorates the quality of food. For example—Remove cream from milk.

(c) Addition of harmful substances to good food endangers health. For example—Metanil yellow used in burfi, laddu, haldi.

What is Adulteration?

The way in which the quality of food is lowered is called adulteration. It can be defined as "lowering the quality of food by adding cheap/inferior substances to of or by removing an important part of it or by presence of harmful substances in the food.

Food adulteration can be incidental or intentional. Intentional adulteration of food is done to make more profit while the incidental adulteration is due to negligence, i.e., some harmful substances getting mixed with food accidentally.

What is an Adulterant ?

An adulterant can be defined as 'any cheap outside item which looks the same as the original item which looks the same as the original foodstuff, which mixed very well with it and is not very easy to detect'. These are: stone, chips, mud balls, grit, bark, twigs and parts of plant, similar seeds, starch, sugar, powdered seeds, san dust.

When is the Food Adultered?

Prevention of Food Adulteration Act, 1954 (PFA) describes the conditions under which the food considered adultered. The act came into force on 1st June 1955, The rules since then have been amended in 1968 and 1973 to safeguard the consumers. Food is considered adulterated:

(a) When the nature, substance and quality differ from what it ought to be.

(b) If it contains injurious ingredients.

(c) If it contains cheaper/inferior substances.

(d) If any constituent has been removed/abstracted partially or wholly from it.

(e) If it is infested with insects/worms etc.

(f) If it is prepared, packed and stored under unsanitary conditions.

(g) If it is obtained from sick/diseased animal.

(h) If it contains poisonous ingredients that are injurious to health.

(i) If it contains unpermitted colour. Food is also considered adulterated if it contains excessive amounts of the permitted colours.

(j) If it contains prohibited preservatives. Food is also considered adulterated if it contains excessive amounts of the permitted preservatives.

(k) If it contains chemically react with the food and makes it poisonous and injurious to health.

(l) If it does not satisfy the prescribed standards laid down by authorities.

Commonly Used Foods and the Adulterants Present

You will now study about the various adulterants

present in the foods commonly used is most households.

Cereals: Stones, grit, mud balls are often present in wheat, rice and bajra. Dry things and stems are also mixed with the cereals to increase the weight.

Pulses: Whole daals often have similar stones and metanil yellow also used to enhance the colour.

Sugar, Honey and Jaggery: May have chalk powder and fine chips as the adulterant present in it. Thick syrup add in honey.

Ghee and Oil: Vanaspati add in pure ghee to make more profits. Cheaper oil mix oil mustard oil.

Milk: Addition of water and removal of cream from milk lower the quality of milk.

Tea and Coffee: Used and coloured tea leaves are the common adulterants responsible for lowing the quality and grade of tea. Coffee is adulterated with chicory beans powder.

Salt and Spices: Salt may be mixed with chalk powder, dirt and stones. Spice powders are often adulterated with excessive amounts of sand, straw, sawdust or cowdung.

Health Hazards of Common Adulterants

Adulterants	*Foods Adulterated*	*Hazards*
Stone, chips, mud grit and sawdust	Cereals, pulses, jaggery and spices	Stomach upset balls, stones can damage teeth and intestine.
Kesari dal	Channa dal, arhar dal, kesari dal powder	Consumption of besan, and moong dal causes paralysis of lower limbs diseases
Metanil yellow	Enhance the colour of dal, besan haldi etc.	They crippling is called lathyrilsm and mainly attacks boys and men between the ages of 5-45 years

Talcum powder Asbestos powder	Pulses are mixed with talcum and asbestos powder	Causing stomach trouble, liver and kidney damage
Argemine oil	Mustard oil help adultered with cheap oil	Stomach upset, kidney stone and stomach cancer
Rhodamine B blindness	Red chillies	Partial and total and hazards of heart.
Mineral oil	Edible oil	Trouble in liver, kidney and spleen. It cannot absorb by body

Detection of Adulterant Present in Foods

Cereals: Should be picked and cleaned before cooking them. The stones, twigs and other plants parts can be seen and picked. Washing of the cereals grains enables one to remove the mud and dirt.

Pulses: Visual check of pulses will enable one to separate the kesari daal from the arhar and chana dals. Put some dal in a test tube. Add water and shake. Add dilute HCl (Hydrochloric acid) and shake. Presence of magenta red colour shows that the dal is adultered with metanil yellow.

Milk and Milk Products: Addition of water and starch, removal cream lower the quality of milk. Transfer milk from one glass to another, milky appearance of the empty glass suggests that the milk is pure. The lactometer test can be done in the laboratory to find out the specific gravity/density of milk. The specific gravity of pure milk is 1.030-1.034. Starch used in khoya, burfi etc.

Tea and Coffee: Iron filing in tea leaves can easily be defected with the help of a magnet. Tamarind seeds also present in coffee. Put some amount of potassium hydroxide solution on top. Emergence of brown colour and coffee particles confirms adulteration.

Salt: Dissolve the sample of salt in a beaker, dirt settle at the base and salt dissolve in water.

Black Pepper: It looks like similar to papaya seeds at casual glance. Papaya seeds have rough surface as black pepper. Papaya seeds are lighter than black pepper.

Protection Against Food Adulteration

Adulteration of commonly used foods in increasing at an alarming pace. The cost of food is forever increasing and the unscrupulous traders are indulging in malpractices to increase their profit margin. You should safeguard yourself from the menace of adulteration in the following ways:

1. Buy from reliable shops only. If you buy from a shop that has reputation and large sales turnover, you will be able to get fresh and good quality stocks.
2. Buy standard and reliable brands of foods for they will be good quality. Look for the standard marks for getting the full value of your money. Standard marks safeguard against food.

Standard Marks of Foods

The Bureau of Indian Standard (BIS) stands guarantee for the quality of products bearing ISI mark. Indian Standards Institution mark ensures that: (a) The quality of foods particularly those affecting health and safety of consumers is superb. (b) The mass produced and mass consumed products confirm to the required standards of quality, safety and durability.

There is a wide range of consumer goods that carry the ISI mark. As a quality conscious consumer you must look for this mark before purchasing anything. A list of the commodities bearing mark is given below :

Air-conditioner, helmets, immersion heater, ceiling fan, ink pen, stone, gas stove, aluminium vessels, cooking range, safety match, refrigeration, door closers, shaving blades, napthalene balls, liquid toilet soap, detergent powder, handloom cotton, bed sheets, sewing thread, vanaspati, baby foods, biscuits, coffee powder, edible, common salt, chewing gum.

Agmark determines the quality and purity of the agricultural products. The word AGMARK is a derivative of agricultural marketing. The quality of the product is assessed on the basis of production, varies size, shape, weight, colour, moisture, fat content and other relevant physical and chemical characteristics. Agmark products are available in grocery stones, super bazaars and departmental stores. Some of the products bearing Agmark are as follows :

Rice, mustard oil, wheat, pure ghee, pulses, butter, gram flour, honey, mangoes, spices, grapes, curry powder, citrus fruits, black pepper powder, coconut oil, eggs, tea, etc.

Look for "Agmark" symbol on the products you purchase next time and be sure about the purity of the product and the quality of your decision.

I. PFA: Prevention of Food Adulteration Act, 1954 controls that the foods and their products are not adulterated.

II. FPO: Stands for Fruit Products Order and was founded by the government of India in 1946 under the defense of India rules. FPO lays down minimum standards relating to the quality of various fruits and vegetables products. The order specifies the standard of sanitation and hygiene to be followed in the factories, besides giving directions regarding packing, marking, and labeling. If the manufacturer does not confirm to these regulations, he is liable to be punished under the provision of the law.

The food bearing marks are:

Jam, baked beans, syrups, jellies, sardines, pickles, marmalade, soap, chutnies, ketchup, squashes.

III. Do not buy loose foodstuffs wherever sealed packets and tins are available. It is easier to adulterate loose food materials than temper with the packet stuff.

IV. Study the label and the standard mark before purchasing the foodstuff. A good label provides the consumer with the following information:

(i) Name of the foodstuffs.
(ii) Ingredients contained.
(iii) Date of manufacturing and date of expiry.
(iv) Name, place and address of manufacturer.
(v) Net contents and cast excluding local taxes.
(vi) Instructions for storage and use.
(vii) Standard mark for quality product.

V. Be quality conscious and sure that you are not being cheated by adulteration. In case you suspect the shopkeeper on the manufacturer of adulating the foodstuff do notify to the concerned authorities for proper action. Public health laboratories test and analyze adulterated foodstuff. These laboratories work under the guidance of central food laboratories. The seller and manufacturer if found guilty can even get life imprisonment. These laboratories are situated at Collate, Pine, My sore and Ghazi bad.

Besides government agencies already mentioned, certain voluntary agencies also contribute to check the menace of adulteration. These are:

(a) Quality control laboratories of food company's, e.g., canning industry.
(b) Quality control laboratories of consumer organizations, e.g., super bazaar.
(c) Private testing laboratories.

Besides the standard marks studies so far, you may have also heard of eco-mark. It is put on products that are environment friendly or eco-friendly. It ensures that the product is biogradable and will not pollute the environment.

Have you seen wool mark? When you see this woolmark on woollen cloth, you can be sure of its quality and purity.

Summary

- The food is considered adulterated when it is mixed with cheap, inferior and harmful substances.
- It is also deemed adulterated when some valuable constituent is removed from it.
- Stone, dirt, dry plant parts, colour starch, and sawdust etc. are the common adulterants present in foods.
- Prevention of Food Adulteration Act (PFA) gives specifications as to when the food is adulterated.
- Adulterated food causes hazards ranging from stomach upset to the impairment of vital functioning of kidney, heart, reproductive and nervous systems.
- Simple tests to defect the adulterant present can be performed at home and in home science laboratory.
- Importance of standard marks for providing protection against adulteration.

Possible Health Hazards of Hawker's School Snacks

Name of the Snacks	*Adulterates*	*Health Hazards*
Aam papad	Dust, insect excreta	Nausea, vomiting
Ice candy	Metanil yellow	Diarrhoea, abdominal pain
Karachi halwa	Metanil yellow	Degeration of testes in males, cancer
Rasgulla	Poisonous colour	Lesions in ritual organ
Sugar coated saunf	Melachite green	Abnormalities in bone, lungs, eyes

Coconut churan	Sawdust	Stomach irritation, mental retardation
Supari	Auramine dirt	Brain damage
Toffee	Soap stone	Stomach cancer
Moong dal	Metanil yellow	Degeneration of testes
Groundnut	Fungus and fungal toxin	Liver damage

11

Food Preparation

Food safety has made headlines in newspapers and magazines lately due to outbreaks of diseases such as hepatitis, *E. coli* infections, and food poisoning, to name a few. Common food poisonings found in humans include *E. coli* 0157:H7, salmonella, campylobacter and listeria. Leaving fresh food and water in the bird's cage for several hours may be the cause of bacterial infections in birds.

In our aviary, wet food is left in cages for approximately 6 hours during the winter months, and for less time during the summer months. We try to maintain a temperature in our aviaries of 70ºF. But it sometimes rises when the outside temperature is above 90ºF. However, we seldom have bacterial problems in our flock.

There are several ways to prepare foods which will help reduce the risk of infectious disease problems in birds:

Wash Your Hands

My veterinarian has told me on more than one occasion that one would be surprised at how effective hand washing with a good antibacterial soap can be against bacteria. I wash my hands several times during preparation of foods for our birds, and especially after handling raw meats or eggs. Hands should be dried with a clean towel or paper towel.

Sanitize Cutting Surfaces and Utensils

We chop vegetables and fruits with a very sharp knife, on a built-in cutting board, both of which are washed and dried thoroughly between foods.

It would be wise to disinfect your cutting surface and utensils daily with a disinfectant, or a mixture of 3 teaspoons of chlorine bleach mixed in 1 gallon of water. (I don't suggest using this bleach mixture around your birds, however, because it may cause eye and lung irritation). Disinfecting is a sanitation practice that is absolutely necessary if raw meat or eggs have been cut on the cutting surface.

Wash Foods

Before foods are cut and served, they are thoroughly washed. Some people use a solution of 1 part Nolvansan liquid to 8 parts water; or 1 teaspoon chlorine bleach (which contains sodium hypochlorite and no phosphorus) in 1 gallon of water. Fruits and vegetables can be soaked for up to 10 minutes, then rinsed thoroughly in another bowl with running water for at least 5 minutes. Be sure to inspect foods thoroughly before washing them to detect mold, overripe or brown spots.

It should go without saying that any meats which are being prepared should be thoroughly washed, whether they are for human or your birds' consumption.

Cook Meats Thoroughly

Any meats we serve our birds, which include turkey, chicken, or beef, must be well cooked.

One caller told me she feeds her birds meats prepared on the barbeque grill cooked medium well-done. I would strongly suggest that if you want to serve ground meat cooked on the grill, to recook it in the microwave, to make absolutely certain the center is well cooked. (*Note*: Cooking the center to well done is applicable only to ground meat. The center of a steak or roast is absolutely free of *E. coli* or other contaminants. Only something the animal consumes can get into the meat or something live which infiltrates, such as trichinosis in pork.

Also, remember that meats should not be served to our birds if they have been left out for any length of time. A good example of this would be turkey that has been left on the table after Thanksgiving dinner, while the participants are visiting.

Of course, food handling is not always the cause of infectious agents found in foods. The *E. coli* bacterium was found in frozen hamburger patties prepared at a meat plant. An outbreak of hepatitis A was traced to strawberries packaged by a company in San Diego, but the frozen strawberries were from Mexico, and used in Michigan. An outbreak of cyclospora (a parasite) was blamed on Guatemalan raspberries.

Though not affecting our birds, another disease outbreak was caused by tainted ice-cream which had been transported by trucks that previously carried raw eggs.

A recent newspaper article reported that on crops, contamination occurs from the use of untreated water for irrigation or fertilizers containing the dangerous organisms. It went on to say that cattle feed may include contaminated animal parts or waste material. It was further reported that Mexico is the primary exporter of vegetables to the United States. The author of this article explained that in one particular town whose crops he observed, the surrounding communities emptied their sewage into the river which supplied the water to irrigate fields of corn.

Mexico is now shipping winter fruits and vegetables which may be contaminated with pesticides or other chemicals. Restrictions on chemicals sprayed on crops are much less stringent south of the border than in the United States. Some foods coming in are hot peppers, watermelons, squash, strawberries, carrots, berries, kiwi, other tropical fruits, and pears. It is a good idea to check packages or signs at the produce counters in grocery stores before purchasing fresh fruits and vegetables. In the past, imported grapes have received bad press due to overuse of chemicals.

Organically grown and prepared foods are very popular for ourselves and our birds, but they are expensive and may be difficult to grow ourselves. Besides, their safety has been questioned because they are often fertilized with manure which could well be contaminated.

Unfortunately, the federal agencies and watchdog groups cannot be expected to inspect and approve every fruit and vegetable we and our birds eat, so it is up to us to determine which foods are safe and healthy, and to educate ourselves about safe food preparation, for the benefit of ourselves and our wards.

12

Food Selection and Storage

Food Quality and Safety

Storage does not improve the quality of any food. The quality of a food will also not decrease significantly during storage as long as the food is stored properly and used within the recommended time frame.

Quality is not the same as safety. A poor-quality food may be safe such as stale cereal, overripe fruit or soured pasteurized milk. An unsafe food may have good quality in terms of appearance and taste, but have a high (unsafe) bacterial count. For example, improperly canned food may contain *Clostridium botulinum*) thus making food unsafe. Or cooked chicken may be placed on a plate that held the raw chicken and become contaminated. The goal of home food storage is to provide both safe and high-quality foods.

Maintaining a food's quality depends on several factors: the quality of the raw product, the procedures used during processing, the way the food is stored and the length of storage. For example, fresh-picked corn will store better than corn that has been in the market for a few days; a tightly folded inside cereal box liner will prevent a ready-to-eat cereal from becoming limp. The recommended storage time takes these factors into consideration.

Since bacteria frequently get into food through careless food handling, keep everything — hands, pantry, shelves and storage containers — clean.

Selection Guidelines

To help assure quality, some products have "open dates" on the package. Product dating is optional on most products. Dates may also be "coded" by the manufacturer and only understood by them. The most commonly used open dates are:

***Sell-by Date*:** This is the last recommended day of sale. The date allows for home storage and use. You will find the date after the statement "sell by (a date)." Breads and baked goods may have "sell-by" dates.

Use-by Date: Tells how long the product will retain top quality after you buy it. You will find this date after statement "Use by." Some packaged goods have "use-by" dates.

***Expiration Date*:** This is the last day the product should be used or eaten. You may find this date after the statement, "Do not use after (date)." Yeast and baking powder have expiration dates.

***Pack Date*:** Canned or packaged foods may have pack dates, which tell you when the product was processed. This does not tell you how long the food will be good.

These are guidelines; if a food is not properly handled, its storage life will be shortened. Follow these tips for purchasing top-quality foods that have been handled safely.

- Look for packages of food that are not torn or broken.
- Canned goods should be free of dents, cracks and bulging lids.
- Refrigerated food should feel cold and frozen food should be frozen solid. Purchase these foods last.

- When shopping, place packaged raw meat, poultry and fish in plastic bags and keep from contact with other foods.
- Take perishable foods home quickly to refrigerate. If travel time will exceed one hour, pack fresh meats in a cooler with ice and keep in the passenger area of the car in warm weather.
- At home, refrigerate perishable food immediately. The "DANGER ZONE" for most food is 40 to 140°F. Bacteria grow most rapidly in this range of temperatures, doubling in number in as little as 20 minutes.

Storage Guidelines

For best results in maintaining product quality practice the rule, FIRST IN, FIRST OUT. This means you use the oldest products first and the newest products later. A good practice in the home is to place the newly purchased products in back of the same products already on the shelf. It may help to write purchase dates on products without "open dates" on the package. Follow recommended storage times for the refrigerator, freezer and pantry (see charts).

Freezer

- Keep freezer temperature at or below 0°F. A good indication of proper temperature is that ice-cream will be frozen solid.
- Use moisture-proof, freezer-weight wrap. Examples are foil, freezer bags and freezer paper. Label and date all packages.
- Food stored beyond the recommended time will be safe to eat, but eating quality (flavour and texture) and nutritive value will be reduced.
- Keep an inventory of freezer contents.

Refrigerator

- Use a thermometer to check temperature; it must be between 34°F and 40°F at all times. Avoid frequently opening the refrigerator door, especially in hot weather.
- Wrapping perishable food prevents the loss of flavour and the mixing of flavour and odors resulting in, for example, onion-flavoured milk.
- Raw meat and poultry should be wrapped securely so they do not leak and contaminate other foods. Place the store packages in a plastic bag or place the package on a plate to contain any juices. Clean up leaks with warm soapy water and sanitize with a solution of 1 teaspoon chlorine bleach to 1 quart water.
- Cooked meats and leftovers should be tightly wrapped to prevent leakage and drying out.

Pantry

- Storage cabinets should be cool and dry. Storage areas near oven ranges, hot water pipes or heating ducts should not be used because heat and moisture can cause a food to lose its quality more rapidly.
- High temperature or humidity may reduce storage time considerably.
- Insect infestation can occur in any home. Susceptible foods include cereals, flour, seeds, baking mixes, spices, candy, dried fruits and dry pet foods. Avoid purchasing damaged packages of foods and keep cupboard shelves clean. Storing food in tightly sealed glass, metal or rigid plastic containers may help.
- Pantry foods will probably be safe beyond recommended storage time, but eating quality (flavour and texture) and nutritive value will be reduced.

Recommended Times for Refrigerator and Freezer Food Storage

Refrigerator and Freezer Foods:

Dairy: Fresh milk 5-7 days – Buttermilk 1-2 weeks–Canned milk (opened) 3-5 days–Yogurt, cottage cheese 7 days–Hard cheese 6-12 weeks 6-12 months–Cheese spreads 3-4 weeks–Ice-cream–2 month.

Eggs: Fresh in shell 3 weeks–Hard-cooked–1 week.

Meats, Frest: Beef roasts, steaks 3-5 days 6-12 months–Ground beef or stew1-2 days 3-4 months–Pork roasts, chops 3-5 days 4-6 months–Sausage 1-2 days 1-2 months Chicken or turkey 1-2 days 9-12 months.

Meats, Cooked: Smoked sausage, whole ham (fully cooked) 7 days 1-2 month sham slices (fully cooked) 3-4 days1-2 months–Hot dogs, luncheon meats (unopened) 2 weeks1-2 months–Hot dogs, luncheon meats (opened) 3-7 days 1-2 months–Cooked, leftover meat 3-4 days 2-3 months–Leftover gravy and meat broth 1-2 days 2-3 months–Cooked, leftover poultry 3-4 days 4-6 months.

Seafood: Fresh lean fish: cod, flounder, trout, haddock, halibut– pollack, perch 1-2 days 4-6 months–Fresh fatty fish: mullet, smelt, salmon, mackerel, bluefish, tuna, swordfish 1-2 days 2-3 months–Live crabs and lobster same day purchased–Live mussels and clams 2-3 days–Live oysters 7-10 days–Mussels and clams, freshly shucked 1-2 days 3-4 months– Oysters, freshly shucked 5-7 days 3-4 months–Scallops, crabmeat, shrimp 2-3 days 3-4 months.

Fruits and Vegetables: Apples1 months 8-12 months–Apricots, avocados, grapes, peaches, pears, plums 3-5 days 8-12 months–Berries, cherries 2-3 days 8-12 months–Grapefruit, lemons, limes, oranges 2 weeks 4-6 months Pineapple 2-3 days 4-6 months Beets, carrots 2 weeks 8-12 months–Beans, broccoli, greens, peas, summer squash 3-5 days 8-12 months –Celery, cabbage, chilies, lettuce, peppers, tomatoes 1 week 8-12 months–Mushrooms 1-2 days 8-12 months.

Pies: Chiffon pie, pumpkin pie 1-2 days 1 month Fruit pie1-2 days. 1 year–Storage here not recommended due to safety or quality issues.

Food Stored in Cool , Dry Pantry (65 to 70°F)

Canned fruits, tomatoes, pickles 12-18 month, scanned meats and vegetables 2-5 years–Home-canned foods 1 year–Fresh root vegetables (onions, potatoes) 1 week at room temperature or 1-3 months at 45–50°F?

The following foods should be stored in the pantry in tightly sealed or airtight containers:

Staples: Nonfat dry milk 1 year,–Pasta 1-2 years, Rice 1 year,– Shortening –2 years–Sugar, granulated indefinitely–Sugar, brown or powdered 18 months Vegetable oil 1 year–White flour 10-15 months–Whole wheat flour 3 months (best in refrigerator or freezer)–Wild rice 6 months.

Packaged Foods: Baking mix (biscuit, cake) 6 months–Cereals 12 months.

Dried Foods: Dried apricots 3 months (refrigerate after opening)–Dried prunes, raisins 9 months (refrigerate after opening) Dried peas and beans 1 year.

Herbs, Spices and Condiments: Salt, cream of tartarindefinitely Ground spices and herbs 2-3 years–Whole spices 4-5 years–Tabasco, vinegar, Worcestershire sauce 30 months.

Beverages (Sealed, Unopened): Bottled water 2-5 years–Juices12-18 months– Soft drinks 8 months.

Miscellaneous: Chocolate 2 years–Chocolate chips, cocoa 18 months–Coffee (canned) 12 months–Nuts (unshelled) 6-12 months–Peanut butter 3-4 months (best refrigerated)–Tapioca 4 years–Tea 18 months.

Bread and Cakes: Store breads and cakes at room temperature. Storing in the refrigerator promotes staling. Use within 3-7 days or freeze.

13

Health

Good health is a vital part of living. Health provides man an instrument to fight disease. But now day's steady progress is made in field of education, medicine, surgery as well as public health. Health is a matter which affect not only each individual but also the community in which we live. An individual keeps fit, he cannot make full use of his life nor can acting community play its proper role in the world. Concept of health is vitally important to all of us and perfect health for community. To achieve this adequate food in necessity of health.

Continuously, day and night the different parts of our body are working as machine. If these go on working smoothly, so the body is to be healthy. If, this natural and normal state it upset or something goes wrong with any function of body, then body becomes ill.

According to World Health Organization (WHO) health as "a state of complete physical, mental and social well being and not merely the absence of disease or infirmity".

Affecting Dimensions of Health or Factor

There are so many factors affecting health, for both the individual and the community. Ill health and unhappiness it causes can be controlled and even prevented. The following factors affect the maintenance of food health.

(i) *Physical*: This means the correct use of the body

mechanism at every stage of life, it means physical fitness. It can be brought about by eating the right kind of found in sufficient quantities along with an adequate amount of exercises and attention to the rules of health.

(ii) *Mental and Emotional:* A mentally unsound person develops physical trouble because mind and body are closely relation. Mental health influenced by emotions like, fear, anger, worry, jay and hatredness. On the other hand, when the mind in happy, good food is an apprehended.

(iii) *Social*: Social factor depends upon its progress, broad mind ness, consideration, thoughtfulness, and sympathy towards other. It influence education, productivity, health and social security.

(iv) *Spiritual:* Due to stress and strain of modern life, is very important to consider this dimension of health. Attention to moral values, ethics, exercises and meditation are same ways of attaining spiritual factor.

Positive Health

An individual who is influenced by above these factors is in a state of complete on positive health. A person is able to line healthy in this environment and depends on the family and community as well. Food is the basic important factor toward maintaining optimum positive health. Lack of proper food causes deficiency diseases. Medicines are needed to cure on promote health and prevent disease.

Human Body Composition

The human body comprises chemical compounds such as water, amino acids (proteins), fatty acids nucleic acids, and carbohydrates. These compounds in turn consist of elements such as carbon, hydrogen, oxygen, nitrogen, and phosphorus, and may or may not contain minerals such as calcium, iron, and zinc. Minerals also ubiquitously occur in the form of salts and electrolytes.

All of these chemical compounds and elements occur in various forms and combinations, both in the human body and in organisms that humans eat.

The human body must necessarily comprise those elements that humans eat and absorb into the bloodstream. The digestive system, except in the unborn fetus, is the first step in helping to make the different chemical compounds and elements in food available for the trillions of cells of the body. In the digestive process of an average adult, about seven litres of liquid, known as digestive juices, exit the internal body and enter the lumen of the digestive tract. The digestive juices help break chemical bonds between ingested compounds as well as modulate the conformation and/or energetic state of the compounds/elements. Yet many compounds/ elements are absorbed into the bloodstream unchanged, though the digestive process helps to release them from the matrix of the foods where they occur. Any unabsorbed matter is eliminated in the feces. Only a minimal amount of digestive juice is eliminated this way; the intestines reabsorb most of it otherwise the body would rapidly dehydrate.

Study in this field must take into careful account the state of the body before ingestion and after digestion as well as the chemical content of both the food and the waste. The specific types of compounds and elements that are absorbed by the body can be determined by comparing the waste to the food. The effect that the absorbed matter has on the body can be determined by finding the difference between the pre-ingestion state and the post-digestion state. The effect may only be discernible after an extended period of time in which all food and ingestion must be exactly regulated and all waste must be analyzed. The number of variables (e.g. 'confounding factors') involved in this type of experimentation is very high. This makes scientifically valid nutritional study very time-consuming and expensive, which accounts for why a proper science of human nutrition is rather new.

In general, eating a variety of fresh, whole (unprocessed) foods has proven hormonally and metabolically favourable compared to eating a monotonous diet based on processed foods. In particular, fresh, whole foods provide higher amounts and a more favourable balance of essential and vital nutrients per unit of energy, resulting in better management of cell growth, maintenance, and mitosis (cell division) as well as of appetite and energy balance. A generally more regular eating pattern (e.g., eating medium-sized meals every 3 to 4 hours) has also proven more hormonally and metabolically favourable than infrequent, haphazard food intake.

Role of Nutrition

The role of nutrition in health was recognized by the ancient Greeks–and probably also much earlier–who advised that food should be one's medicine. Especially eastern cultures have for more than two thousand years used certain foods (e.g., herbs) as remedy. Clearly these early insights were based on simple observations that *nutrition*–aside from the obvious need to eat sufficient energy–has a direct effect on the health of the organism.

In the 18th century, many sailors on long journeys died from scurvy; indeed, some naval ships lost more men through illness than through enemy action. The cause of this was not understood until it was discovered that adding fresh limes to the ship's supply of preserved food seemed to boost the sailors' resistance to the illness and resulted in fewer deaths. The existence of separate compounds/elements in food that are essential for survival had been discovered, and this discovery of Vitamin C which prevents scurvy spurred the search for other so-called 'essential nutrients'.

In the latter half of the 20th century, technological developments and a world wide epidemic of lifestyle related diseases has spurred detailed research into the specific health effects of different foods. For example, in the years following the Second World War, the prevalence of heart disease in western countries began escalating and came under the scrutiny of nutritional researchers around the world, especially in the USA. An increased intake of fat and cholesterol was thought to be a major cause, but later epidemiologic research has demonstrated that the prevalence of heart disease has continued to increase markedly despite a significant decrease in fat intake. Further, none of the performed randomized controlled trials assessing the role of dietary cholesterol or saturated fat in heart disease convincingly support the hypotheses that dietary cholesterol (unoxidized) and saturated fat (from fresh, whole foods) in and of themselves promote heart disease.

Later research has revealed the potential adverse effects on (heart) health of trans fatty acids, which were introduced to the human diet large scale with the new technology of lipid hydrogenation. Partially hydrogenated oils were added to many processed foods and helped make possible the production of solid margarine from cheap liquid vegetable oils, and helped increase the shelf-life of many foods. In the late 90's the harmful effects of excess trans fatty acids in the diet came into the attention of the public and governments began restricting or banning its use.

While one 'camp' of researchers focused on the hypothetical benefits of reduced intake of fat and cholesterol, another 'camp' emphasized the possible benefits (initially for diabetics) of reducing intake of carbohydrates and thereby preventing excess blood sugar raise and stimulation of the fundamental, all-important hormone insulin. In the early 80's, researchers began to systematically measure the amount of sugar in subjects' blood before and after consumption of foods containing a standard amount of digestible carbohydrate (e.g. 50 grams). The resulting comparable values of the blood sugar raising potential of different carbohydrate foods are ranked in the Glycemic Index. In general, the Glycemic Index demonstrates that eating processed, carbohydrate-dense foods (higher GI) results in a higher blood sugar raise and insulin release than does eating whole, unprocessed carbohydrate-containing foods (lower GI). In more recent years, researchers have focused more on the glycemic load which factors in the amount of carbohydrate eaten, whereas the Glycemic Index only compares the blood sugar raising potential of foods with a set amount of carbohydrate (i.e. eating large amounts of low GI foods can result in a higher blood sugar raise and insulin stimulation than eating small amounts of high GI foods).

The recent advances in molecular biology and gene technology, for example with the use of 'knock-out' animal models where specific genes are inactivated, have enabled a more informative study of how nutrition 'communicates' with our genes and thus with the chief metabolic hormones. Since the Human Genome Project was completed, the focus has shifted towards study of the proteome. The study of hormones and other cell-to-cell signalling molecules is receiving special attention.

The previous mechanistic view of food merely as fuel thus falls short. Foods and their diverse components are capable of affecting the control of metabolism directly via hormones and genes, to the effect that different foods can for example affect energy expenditure to varying degrees, also when energy intake is constant.

Nutrition and Health

The health can be brought about by an imbalance of nutrients, producing either an excess or deficiency which in turn affects body functioning in a cumulative manner. In addition, as mentioned, the type and amount of foods we eat affect the body's hormonal environment directly, and a persistent intake of (a certain amount of) certain foods may induce hormonal imbalance and thereby disease. Moreover, because most nutrients are, in some way or the other, involved in cell-to-cell signalling (e.g. as building block or part of a hormone), deficiency or excess of various nutrients affects hormonal function also indirectly. Thus, because they largely regulate the expression of genes, hormones represent a link between nutrition and how our genes are expressed, i.e., our phenotype. The strength and nature of this link are continually under investigation, but observations especially in recent years have demonstrated a pivotal role for nutrition in hormonal activity and function and therefore in health.

Mineral and vitamin deficiency may yield symptoms of diminishing health such as goitre, scurvy, osteoporosis, weak immune system, disorders of cell metabolism, certain forms of cancer, symptoms of premature aging, and poor psychological health (including eating disorders).

As of 2005, twelve vitamins and about the same number of minerals are recognized as 'essential nutrients', meaning that they must be consumed and absorbed–or, in the case of Vitamin D, alternatively synthesized via UVB radiation - to prevent deficiency symptoms and death. Certain vitamin-like substances found in foods, such as carnitine, have also been found essential to survival and health, but these are not strictly 'essential' to eat because the body can produce them from other compounds. Moreover, thousands of different phytochemicals have recently been discovered in food (particularly in fresh vegetables), which have many discovered and yet to be discovered properties including antioxidant activity. Other essential nutrients include essential amino acids, choline and the essential fatty acids.

In addition to sufficient intake, an appropriate

balance of essential fatty acids–omega-3 and omega-6 fatty acids–has been discovered to be crucial for maintaining health. Both of these unique 'omega' long-chain unsaturated fatty acids are substrates for a class of eicosanoids known as prostaglandins). Alpha-linolenic acid (LNA) serves as the building block for the less-inflammatory PGE3 series of prostaglandins, whereas linoleic acid (LA) (and specifically its product, AA) serves as the building block for either the PGE1 (anti-inflammatory) or the PGE2 (pro-inflammatory) series. (The omega-6 fatty acid LA is the building block for the omega-6 fatty acid AA, but AA can also be obtained directly in the diet). The conversions of AA into the respective prostaglandins (PGE1/PGE2) have importantly been discovered to be under hormonal control, as certain hormones such as insulin and glucagon regulate the function of the enzymes responsible for the conversions. Because different types and amounts of food eaten/absorbed affect insulin, glucagon and other hormones to varying degrees, not only the amount of omega-3 versus omega-6 eaten but also the general composition of the diet is now known to determine health implications in relation to essential fatty acids, inflammation (e.g. immune function) and mitosis (i.e. cell division).

Several lines of evidence indicate lifestyle-induced insulin malfunction, referred to as insulin resistance, as a decisive factor in many disease states. Researchers have for long assumed that overfatness/obesity causes insulin resistance, which in turn causes type 2 diabetes (virtually all obese and diabetic individuals have marked insulin resistance). More recent evidence has however demonstrated that insulin resistance may well be the cause of overfatness/obesity as well as type 2 diabetes and possibly other lifestyle-related diseases. For example, it has been demonstrated that appropriate exercise, more regular food intake and reducing glycemic load all can reverse insulin resistance in overfat individuals, which means that lifestyle rather than the fact of being fat promotes insulin resistance.

Nonetheless, overfatness can unfavourably alter hormonal and metabolic status seemingly especially via the hormone leptin, and a vicious cycle may occur in which insulin/leptin resistance and overfatness aggravate one another. There is debate to what extent different dietary factors, such as intake of processed carbohydrates, total protein-, fat-, and carbohydrate intake, intake of trans fatty acids, and low intake of micronutrients, contribute to develop insulin and leptin resistance. Most importantly, insulin and leptin resistance are both strongly linked to chronic inflammation, which in turn is strongly linked to a variety of adverse developments such as arterial microinjuries and clot formation (i.e. heart disease) and over-expressed cell division (i.e. cancer).

A persistent high intake of processed carbohydrate-dense foods (high glycemic load) resulting in repeatedly high release of insulin and leptin seems to readily make cells less responsive to both of these crucial hormones (perhaps especially in combination with high intake of saturated fat/trans fatty acids and sedentary living). This type of negative feedback is ubiquitous in any biological system, all of which depend on appropriate hormonal regulation for survival and proper function. However, certain cell types appear to more readily become resistant to the effects of certain hormones (e.g. insulin, leptin) than others; certain fat cells (e.g. abdominal subcutaneous fat) may respond well to the fat-storing signal of insulin while other cells fail to properly receive/transduce the signal meant to induce important cellular and systemic effects. Why certain cells develop resistance to certain signalling molecules remains unclear, but it seems plausible that hormone resistance serves to protect cells from excess circulating amounts of the given hormone. Analogous to the way modern man-made pollution may potentially overwhelm the environment's ability to maintain homeostasis, the recent explosive introduction of high Glycemic Index–and processed foods into the human diet may potentially overwhelm the body's ability to maintain homeostasis and health (as evidenced by, for example, the obesity epidemic).

Antioxidants are another recent discovery. As cellular metabolism/energy production requires oxygen, potentially damaging (e.g. mutation causing) compounds known as radical oxygen species or free radicals may form. For normal cellular maintenance, growth, and division, these free radicals must be sufficiently neutralized by antioxidant compounds, such as certain vitamins (Vitamin C, Vitamin E, Vitamin K and the aforementioned phytochemicals as well as other compounds, some of which the body itself produces. Different antioxidants are now known to function in a cooperative network, e.g. Vitamin C can reactivate free radical-containing glutathione or Vitamin E by accepting the free radical itself, and so on.

It is now also known that the human digestion system contains a population of a range of bacteria which are essential to digestion, and which are also affected by the food we eat. The role and significance of the intestinal bacterial flora is under investigation.

It is now commonly accepted amongst the medical profession that a diet high in fresh fruit and vegetables but low in animal fat helps to prevent heart disease and cancer.

Nutrition and Longevity

Lifespan is somehow related to the amount of food energy consumed: this was first systematically investigated in the seminal study by Weidruch, et al. (1986). A pursuit of this principle of caloric restriction followed, involving research into longevity of those who reduced their food energy intake while attempting to optimize their micronutrient intake. Perhaps not surprisingly, some people found that cutting down on food reduced their quality of life so considerably as to negate any possible advantages of lengthening their lives. However, a small set of individuals persists in the lifestyle, going so far as to monitor blood lipid levels and glucose response every few months.

This has set researchers off on a line of study which presumes that it is not low food energy consumption which increases longevity. Instead, longevity may depend on an efficient fat processing metabolism, and the consequent long term efficient functioning of our organs free from the encumbrance of accumulating fatty deposits. Thus, longevity may be related to maintained insulin sensitivity. However, several other factors including low body temperature seem to promote longevity also and it is unclear to what extent each of them contribute.

14

Water

Our bodies are about two-thirds water, and we need to ensure that we keep up this balance in order to remain healthy. That's why it is recommended that you drink at least eight glasses of water every day. This will keep all your organs hydrated so that they can function properly, and water also helps to flush toxins and other impurities out of your body. Water serves many other crucial functions including: respiration, digestion, metabolism, body temperature regulation and excretion. Water is also responsible for dissolving and transporting nutrients through the body. Only oxygen is more important to sustaining human life than water. So, drink a tall glass of water and stay healthy.

Water of Life

Water is the very stuff of life and we need lots of it. Humans lose about 10 cups (about 2.4 liters) of fluid a day in sweat, urine, exhaled air and bowel movements. To replace that and keep a fluid balance, you need to drink between eight and 12 glasses of water a day, regardless of the weather. Caffeinated and alcoholic beverages don't count, since they are actually dehydrating and increase urine output.

Apart from those people who suck on a pump bottle all day long, it is likely that most people don't drink sufficient water. Fortunately, food makes up some of our water intake. A slice of bread, for instance, is 38 per cent water and a medium baked potato with skin is 70 per cent. In the average diet, solid foods provide between three and four cups of water daily.

Function of Water

It is generally accepted that water is needed to regulate body temperature, transport nutrients and other substances throughout the body, carry away waste and moisten, lubricate and cushion the body from injury. Since every function of the body is monitored and pegged by the efficient flow of water, "water distribution is the only way of making sure that not only an adequate amount of water, but its transported elements (hormones, chemical messengers and nutrients), first reach the more vital organs".

Need of water

The need for water starts early, says Batman. "Morning sickness of the mother is a thirst signal of both the fetus and the mother." Batman argues that Alzheimer's disease is primarily caused by brain cell dehydration. In a dehydrated state many functions of the brain cells begin to get lost, such as the transport system that delivers neurotransmitters to the nerve endings.

Water, it seems, will not only enable you to retain your marbles, but also keep you spry. There is nothing better for rheumatoid arthritis than water, says Batman. Since the cartilage surfaces of bones in a joint contain much water, dehydration will have the effect of reducing lubrication in the joints and causing pain. Since 75 per cent of the weight of the upper body is supported by the water volume stored in the disc core of our vertebrae, sufficient water will also ease back pain.

But wait, there's more. Migraine, argues Batman, can also be prevented by regular intakes of water. Water shortage increases the potential for hypertension because the body copes with chronic dehydration by taking about eight per cent water from blood volume. This causes some capillaries to close down, says Batman, causing hypertension. "Essential hypertension should be treated with an increase in water intake." Higher cholesterol levels also denote dehydration, since excess cholesterol is manufactured in the cell membrane to protect it against dehydration. "If you do not drink water before you eat a meal, the process of food digestion will take its toll on the body. Water will have to be poured on the food in the stomach for proteins to break down and separate into the basic composition of amino acids. In the intestine, more water will be required to process the food ingredients and send them to the liver."

Batman recommends taking one glass of water half an hour before breakfast, lunch and dinner and a similar amount two and a half hours after each meal. "This is the very minimum amount of water your body needs." Two more glasses should be taken before going to bed - water can also help you sleep. "Try drinking a glass of water and then putting a pinch of salt on your tongue. My personal experience and observation in others have shown that one begins to fall asleep after a few minutes. In my estimation, this combination alters the rate of electrical discharge in the brain and induces sleep."

When the body is well hydrated, one or two glasses of water "before the event" will help in achieving a firmer and sustained erection in men and joy of participation in women.

15

Food Hygiene

Introduction

A major chink of one's income is spending on food alone. Safe food is needed by every living organism to grow, keep healthy and have a productive life span. Food can become unfit for consumption at various stages, i.e., from harvesting, storing, cooking, serving to consuming. As such it is of utmost importance that safety of person, place and food is maintained.

Safe Food Consumption

The food handlers need to exercise utmost care with handling food for the family right from the time it is purchased, stored, cooked, processed and served.

Safety measures should be kept in mind while purchasing foods. One should keep in mind the needs of the family and the storage facilities available at home. The quantity purchased will be dependent upon the availability of money and storage space.

Buy food materials from reliable shop. This way you are assured of the cost, quality and freshness of foods purchased. It is economical to buy from super bazaars and cooperative stores. Buy from clean and hygienic stores, cooperatives and bazaars.

Some foods are eaten mean while most others are cooked. Appropriate methods of cooking ensure availability of maximum nutrients. Safe handling of food is essential to check the infection and spoilage of food during cooking and processing.

Serving of food is done by the lady of the house. At times the kitchen helpers also do this job. The health and hygiene standards of food handlers and hygiene should be high. This ensures that only safe food is consumed by the family.

Definition of Food Hygiene

Food gets contaminated when carelessly handled. The bacteria and other toxic materials may find entry into your system through improper and in sanitary handling of food. You must eat food that is free from disease carrying germs and harmful substances to keep well.

Food hygiene can be defined as "the safe handling of food in a way that will keep if safe and free from all contaminants".

Factors Affecting the Safety of Food at Home

Safety of food is a result of all the following factors put together. Any shortcoming in the functioning of one will have a direct influence, on all other factors:

(a) Cleanliness in the kitchen.

(b) Hygienic handling of food.

(c) Personal hygiene.

(a) Cleanliness in the Kitchen

(i) The kitchen should be well lighted and well-ventilated. Few hours of relight in the kitchen will remain dampness besides killing some of the bacteria. A well ventilated kitchen does not smell of food odours. Insects and pests hid in dark dingy kitchen. A dry, well lighted and clean kitchen will keep insects and pest away.

(ii) Kitchen should be fly proof and hence have nest on its doors and windows.

(iii) The dustbin should have liner and be emptied out each day. Have you noticed the, dustbins lined with plastic in some eating places. The waste can be conveniently disposed of and the dustbin is easy to keep clean.

(iv) The kitchen work surface and floors should be easy to maintain and clean. Remove all food scraps immediately. It keep cockroaches and rodents away.

(v) Plenty of hot and cold water should be available for cooking, cleaning food and utensils.

(vi) Keep kitchen clothe/dusters clean. Wash them with good detergent and rinse well.

(vii) Kitchen should have a well organized storage space.

(b) Hygienic Handling of Food

(i) No dirt and disease germs get into the food she is serving to the family.

(ii) Do not leave the food uncovered. Dust, dirt and flies can spoil your food. Always use a cake cover.

(iii) If you have boils on your hands make sure you don't handle the food. Boils have staphylocoees bacteria, the toxins present in staphylocoee bacteria affect the gastro intestinal tract but do not enter the blood stream.

(iv) It is unhygienic to cough and sneeze on food. These bacteria pose health hazards and the infected food can cause sickness to all those who consume this food.

(v) It is a good practice to subject the food to visual inspection. Remove all stones twigs, worms, meevil and infested foods. Rotten and spoilt food should be discarded for safety measures.

(vi) Wash your food well to remove dirt, excessive insecticides and pesticides.

(vii) Cook food thoroughly and for sufficient time to ensure destruction of most bacteria. Pressure cooking is best.

(viii) The left over food should be stored in clean container in the fridge.

(c) Personal Hygiene

(i) Wash your hands with a good soap before and after handling food.

(ii) You should tie your hair to avoid shedding then in your food.

(iii) Tasting food with the Liddell and then returning to same cooking pot is a bad habit. So avoid it.

(iv) Avoid walking into the kitchen with dirty feet/ shoes/chappals and clothing.

(v) Sick individual should not be allowed in the kitchen.

(vi) Wear a clean apron and protect your clothing and yourself.

The Detergent in Your Diet

Detergent get rid of grease and food residues from your utensils but they leave behind injurious residues.

The liquid detergents consist of soluble detergents in water. The detergent used is a sulphonate (Alpha Olefinsulphonate)–AOS the active agent is a liquid detergent makeup 15 to 20 per cent of the product.

The scouring powders contain less than 1 to 3 per cent of AOS. The scouring powders generally contain soda ash which enhances the cleaning action.

It is not easy to rid utensils of residual detergent. Since the abrasive is soluble in water, it is retained on the utensil surface along with the active detergent. Studies carried out at the industrial toxicology research center at Luck now have shown that more than 10 rinses may be needed to completely remove traces of the detergent.

A study of liquid detergent in UK suggests that 50-60 mg of the active detergent may be "eaten" by an adult each day. Babies also ingest it through feeding bottles cleaned with detergents.

Scouring powders contain proportionately less of the active ingredients. While no studies have been done on these powders—an informed estimate by experts is that the average daily consumption from them would be around long.

16

Food Borne Illness

What is Foodborne Illness?

Food borne illness often shows itself as flu-like symptoms such as nausea, vomiting, diarrhea or fever, so many people may not recognize that the illness is caused by bacteria or other pathogens on food. The onset of symptoms may not occur for two or more days after the contaminated food was eaten. Thousands of types of bacteria are naturally present in our environment, but not all bacteria cause disease in humans. For example, some bacteria are used beneficially in making cheese and yogurt.

Bacteria that cause disease are called "pathogens." When certain pathogens enter the food supply, they can cause food borne illness. Only a few types cause millions of cases of food borne illness each year. Most cases of food borne illness can be prevented. Proper cooking or processing of food destroys bacteria.

Age and physical condition place some persons at higher risk than others, no matter what type of bacteria is implicated.

Infants are at greatest risk from any pathogen. Some persons may become ill after ingesting only a few harmful bacteria; others may remain symptom free after ingesting thousands. The following factors make controlling food borne pathogens particularly challenging. Consumers do not always take time to wash hands and utensils or thaw meats properly.

Emerging pathogens demand even greater food safety vigilance than what was required in previous generations. The food supply has become global with many different countries supplying food products to the U.S. More food is prepared and consumed away from home. Also, an increasing amount of food prepared away from the home is then taken home for consumption, thus creating new opportunities for mishandling.

At the same time, bacteria already recognized as sources of food borne illness have found new modes of transmission. While many illnesses from occur from eating undercooked ground beef, these bacteria have also been traced to other foods, such as salami, raw milk, lettuce and unpasteurized apple cider.

Campylobacter Jejuni

These bacteria are the most common cause of diarrhea.

Sources: Raw and undercooked meat and poultry, raw milk and untreated water.

Symptoms: Fever, headache and muscle pain followed by diarrhea (sometimes bloody), abdominal pain and nausea that appear two to five days after eating; may last seven to 10 days.

Listeria Monocytogenes

This organism causes listeriosis, a serious disease for pregnant women, newborns and adults with a weakened immune system.

Sources: Soil and water. It has been found in cheese; raw milk; improperly processed ice cream; raw and undercooked meat; poultry and seafood; and raw, leafy vegetables.

Symptoms: Fever, chills, headache, backache, sometimes abdominal pain and diarrhea that appear 12 hours to three weeks after eating contaminated food. Later more serious illness may develop in at-risk patients (meningitis or spontaneous abortion in pregnant women); sometimes just fatigue.

E. Coli

This bacterium can produce a deadly toxin.

Sources: Meat, especially undercooked or raw hamburger, raw milk, unpasteurized apple juice or cider, uncooked fruits and vegetables, contaminated water, or person to person contact.

Symptoms: Diarrhea or bloody diarrhea, abdominal cramps, nausea, and malaise; can begin two to five days after food is eaten, lasting about eight days. Some, especially the very young, have developed Hemolytic Uremic Syndrome (HUS) that causes acute kidney failure. A similar illness, thrombotic thrombocytopenic purpura (TTP), may occur in older adults.

Salmonella

This group of organisms is the second most common cause of food borne illness. It is responsible for millions of cases of food borne illness a year.

Sources: Raw and uncooked poultry and meat, raw milk and dairy products, seafood, fruits and vegetables, improper handling of food.

Symptoms: Stomach pain, diarrhea, nausea, chills, fever and headache usually appear eight to 72 hours after eating; may last one to two days.

How Bacteria Get in Food

Bacteria may be present on products when you purchase them, such as raw meat, poultry, seafood, eggs or produce. Foods, including safely cooked, ready-to-eat foods, can become cross-contaminated with bacteria transferred from raw products, meat juices or other contaminated products or from poor personal hygiene.

Suspected Foodborne Illness

Preserve the Evidence: If a portion of the suspect food is available, wrap it securely, mark "Danger" and refrigerate it. Save all the packaging materials, such as cans or cartons. Write down the food type, the date and time consumed and when the onset of symptoms occurred. Save any identical unopened products.

Seek Treatment as Necessary: If the victim is in an "at risk" group, or if symptoms persist or are severe (such as bloody diarrhea, excessive nausea and vomiting or high temperature), seek medical care immediately.

Preventing Foodborne Illness

Clean: Wash hands and surface often. Bacteria can spread throughout the kitchen and get on to cutting boards, knives, sponges and counter tops. Wash hands in hot soapy water before preparing food and after using the bathroom, changing diapers and handling pets. For best results, consumers should use warm water to moisten their hands and then apply soap and rub their hands together for 20 seconds before rinsing thoroughly. Wash cutting boards, knives, utensils and counter tops in hot soapy water after preparing each food item and before going on to the next one. Use plastic or other nonporous cutting boards. Cutting boards should be run through the dishwasher — or washed often in hot soapy water — after use.

Consider using paper towels to clean up kitchen surfaces. Or, if using cloth towels, consumers should wash them often in the hot cycle of the washing machine.

Separate: Don't cross-contaminate. Cross-contamination is how bacteria spread from one food product to another.

This is especially true for raw meat, poultry and seafood. Keep these foods and their juices away from ready-to-eat foods. Separate raw meat, poultry and seafood from other food. Store raw meat, poultry and seafood on the bottom shelf of the refrigerator so juices don't drip onto other foods.

If possible, use one cutting board for raw meat products and another for salads and other foods that are ready to be eaten.

Always wash cutting boards, knives and other utensils with hot soapy water after they come in contact with raw meat, poultry and seafood.

Never place cooked food on a plate that previously held raw meat, poultry or seafood.

Cook: Cook to proper temperatures. Foods are properly cooked when they are heated for a long enough time and at a high enough temperature to kill the harmful bacteria that causes food borne illness.

Use a meat thermometer, which measures the internal temperature of cooked meat and poultry, to make sure that the meat is cooked all the way through.

Cook roasts and steaks to a least 145°F. Whole poultry should be cooked to 180°F for doneness.

Cook ground meat, where bacteria can spread during grinding, to at least 160°F. Information from the Centers for Disease Control and Prevention (CDC) links eating undercooked, pink ground beef with a higher risk of illness. If a thermometer is not available, do not eat ground beef that is still pink inside.

Cook eggs until the yolk and white are firm, not runny. Don't use recipes in which eggs remain raw or only partially cooked.

Cook fish until it is opaque and flakes easily with a fork.

Make sure there are no cold spots in food (where bacteria can survive) when cooking in a microwave oven. For best results, cover food, stir and rotate for even cooking. If there is no turntable, rotate the dish by hand once or twice during cooking.

Bring sauces and gravy to a boil when reheating. Heat other leftovers thoroughly to 165°F.

Chill: Refrigerate promptly. Bacteria multiply rapidly between 40°F and 140°F. Refrigerate foods quickly because cold temperatures keep most harmful bacteria from growing and multiplying. Public health officials recommend setting the refrigerator at 34 to 38°F and the freezer unit at 0°F and occasionally checking these temperatures with an appliance thermometer.

Refrigerate or freeze perishables, prepared food and leftovers within two hours.

Never defrost (or marinate) food on the kitchen counter. Use the refrigerator, cold running water or the microwave.

Divide large amounts of leftovers into small, shallow containers for quick cooling in the refrigerator.

With poultry and other stuffed meats, remove the stuffing and refrigerate it in a separate container.

Don't pack the refrigerator. Cool air must circulate to keep food safe.

SECTION-B
CHILD STUDY

17

Developmental Chart

Child development refers to how a child becomes able to do more complex things as they get older. Development is different than growth. Growth only refers to the child getting bigger in size. When we talk about normal development, we are talking about developing skills like:

- **Gross Motor:** Using large groups of muscles to sit, stand, walk, run, etc., keeping balance, and changing positions.
- **Fine Motor:** Using hands to be able to eat, draw, dress, play, write, and do many other things.
- **Language:** Speaking, using body language and gestures, communicating, and understanding what others say.
- **Cognitive:** Thinking skills: including learning, understanding, problem-solving, reasoning, and remembering.
- **Social:** Interacting with others, having relationships with family, friends, and teachers, cooperating, and responding to the feelings of others.

Milestones

Developmental milestones are a set of functional skills or age-specific tasks that most children can do at a certain age range.

Assessment

Assessing your child's development is a team

effort. Pediatrician may also use developmental screening in the office. Screening involves a series of questions and observations that gets at child's ability to perform certain age-appropriate tasks.

Growth and Development

Growth and development are refer to the various aspects of an children overall performance. The various aspects are as follows:

(a) Physical development
(b) Emotional development
(c) Muscular development
(d) Cognitive development
(e) Social development
(f) Language development
(g) Moral development.

(a) Physical Development: It refers to changes in height and weight and the associated changes in shape and size of the child.

There are changes in the body proportions as well. The approximate weight of an Indian child at birth 2.5 kg. The initial doubles by the time the child in 6 months of age. The birth weight triples by the time the child is one year old. At two and three years, the child weights approximately 12 kg and 14 kg respectively.

The average height of an Indian baby at birth is 50 cms. Do you know-how much a child grows in the first year of life? A one year old baby is 20-25 cms more than his/her height at birth two years old child measures 82-85 cms in height. Hereafter the child grow by approximately 8-10 cms per year.

In the fetal state the hands and legs are small and the trunk is like a bag. The head is ¼the body size. The legs and hazards given at a faster rate during infancy.

Consequently the body proportion show considerable improvement as an be seen in the diagram. Development of teeth is an important aspect of physical growth. The human beings get two sets of teeth in life, (a) The primary set/baby/baby teeth/milk teeth, (b) The Permanent teeth, i.e., 20 teeth.

Muscular Development

The bones become strong with calcium deposits. The muscles attached to bones facilitate movement. Do you remember the different kinds of muscles? The muscles become bigger and stronger with age. Muscles enables children to perform tougher jobs with each passing year. The full potential is reached by adolescence.

Physical and muscular developments are together referred to as motor development, toilet control develops with physical and muscular development, mothers should ensure to keep the baby clean and dry. Toilet training can be initiated as early as six months of age. The child can be made to sit an the specially designed toilet seat at regular intervals.

Children are in total control of bowel movement and urination by the time 2 to 2½ years old. They are non ready to go to play schools.

Characteristics

Age 0 to 3 Years

1st Month: The child starts holding head from the age of one month onwards, neck of infants is hardly visible because the skin folds cover it.

Second Month: 2 months old baby an raise his/her chest and head while lying on the abdomen.

Third Month: However, he/she misses to hold the object because of inadequate focusing of vision. Neck starts being visible from 3 months.

4th-5th Month: Children start sitting and complete head control, grasp small objects hold blacks, use specific fingers, thumb to hold play material.

6th Month: Independently sit in a chair grasp objects. They can hold bottle on cup to their mouth for drinking mater and mils.

7th Month: Child's ability to sit independently is remarkable. Infant capable of shifting from lying position to sitting and back again to lying.

8th-9th: Month Children start using legs to move around in their "walker". The child tires to stand by holding the objects in his/her environment, i.e., table, chair etc.

10-12 Month: The child feels happy to stand and hold hands of parents and siblings. He/she tires to take a ten steps with their help.

Age 1-2 years: Child has total control to sit and walk independently.

Age 2-3 years: Motor development shows considerable improvement an account of physical and muscular activity, children can learn and play, jump, playing football, more grasping power.

Social Development

Infants do not show interest in their environment. They are quite content when fed and kept clean and dry. As the child germs he/she starts noticing and recognizing the mother and all those around him/her in the home. Ability to notice others marks the onset of social development.

Characteristics

Age 0-3 Months: They are happy as long as they are fed and clean. They starts recognizing sounds. They start responding by smiling.

Age 4-6 Months: The infants become more social

now. They notice the individuals around then.

Age 7-9 Months: The bonds between the infant and the mother or mother fingers are stronger during this period. They can differentiate between lone and scolding.

Age 10-18 Months: These children indulge in individual play and have very little interaction with other children.

Age 1½to 3 years: The feedings to possession are strong to the extent that the child wants the mother's in divided attention.

Emotional Development

Joy, anger, fear and happiness are some of the emotions that can be noticed even among small children. The emotions are simple reactions that suggests pleasure and displeasure. Sucking at mother's breast, rocking and holding the baby make the child happy. Sudden load noise and wet diapers cause fear and make the child cry. The emotional expressions change with age.

Characteristics

Age 0-3 Months: Children feel distressed when hungry and wet. They feel delighted when talked to in soft tones. They express their feeling by crying and smiling.

Age 4-6 Months: Children showing anger when they are met, hungry and denote find mother around them.

Age 7-9 Months: The development of bonds between mother, child show affection, emotion is expressed by hugging, cuddling.

Age 10-18 Months: Children are worry of strangers, they get scared, they fear the absence of mother.

Age 1½-3 Years: The child becomes jealous of the siblings when the mother attends to their needs.

Cognitive Development

Cognitive development refers to the process of learning and understanding. It is connected with the function of the brain. If you ask a small child fire his/her rattle to you, in all probability you will have no reaction because the child has not understood you. The cognition development of with age. Cognition leads to development of language amongst infants.

Characteristics

Age 0-3 Months: The child satisfy hunger by sucking distinctively. The child circles and the mother feeds the baby.

Age 4-6 Months: Cognition takes time to develop whatever is held by the child is take to the mouth and sucking starts.

Age 7-12 Months: Children development curiosity in this stage. It is very apparent that cognition is modifying child's behaviour.

Age of 1-3 years: The child comes crying to the mother that he/she has been hit by the table. It the tricycle is damaged he/she may force the mother to tie a bandage around its handle, that means child's cognition is developing.

Language Development

Little infants can only produce gurgling and cooing sounds. As they give the babies start making short and simple word sounds like Ma-ma, Ta-tȧ, Cha-cha, Ba-ba, and Pa-pa, etc. This starts the language development which improves with age and repetitive use.

Characteristics

Age 0-3 Months: The only sound that the child can produce is of "crying". By crying they communicate to their mother that they are heavy on well.

Age 4-6 Months: The children of this age group start producing flat "a-a" sounds. Gradually the child starts producing various sounds like pa, ma, ta ba, na and so on.

Age 7-9 Months: The child now produces double flat sounds like baba, mama late, rana and papa etc.

Age 10-12 Months: The children now start speaking in simple sentences. A child who say's "babi-ball" or "babi doll" actually means "baby's" ball and baby's doll."

Moral Development

Small children do not have the ability to discriminate between good and bad or right and wrong. Parents, siblings and family members are the role models for the small child. As the cognitive development improves the child learns to discriminate between good and bad. This starts the moral development of the child at home. It is thus important that the elders around the child show good behaviour.

The various aspects of growth and development occurs at the same time resulting in the overall development of the child.

18

Feeding of the Baby

Food for Infant

Babies are fed with mother's milk, cow's milk, buffalo's milk, goat's milk, donkey's milk or camel's milk. Now, in modern times we have artificial tinned milk for baby like Glaxco, Lactogen-I, Amul etc. Mother's milk undoubtedly the ideal food for the baby where the mother is unable to feed the child nurses are employed at that time, otherwise cows milk is common substitute for the baby.

Breast Feeding

Once the child is born he is separated from the mother and his nourishment has to be provided separately. But this nourishment should be put into the child's mouth to be taken in an digested. From birth there are three available methods of feeding:

1. Breast feeding.
2. Artificial feeding.
3. Combined feeding.

The mother should consider the situation and decide which of the feeding is to be adopted. Breast milk designed by nature from this stage onward until weaning is known as breast milk. Breast milk is natures food for the baby and is the simplest and easiest way to feed the baby.

It is the birth right of every baby to be breast fed. Mothers milk is the best food for any baby. It is most easily digested and is always sterile. Most mothers can produce enough milk for their babies if they observe proper hygiene and had good diet during pregnancy. Mothers milk is the most desirable. A wet nurse is usually unsatisfactory because there is danger of some infectious diseases. Bottle feeding is often necessary and if properly done can very satisfactory and give excellent result.

When Start Breast Feeding

The mother should start feeding as soon as the baby I hungry. It was earlier believed that the babies should be given only sterile water or glucose water during the first day. But now paediatrians believe that the baby should be put to the breast as soon as possible, even in the delivery room. Putting the baby to suck soon after the delivery even if there is no milk in the breast just the has been found to be of great value in successful breast feeding and for the mother child relation ship. The nourishment the baby gets for the first day is not milk but a watery fluid, rich in immunologist called *Colostrum.* It is also contains protein more than mother's milk. But less fats and carbohydrates. Therefore babies who are entirely breast fed rarely get to infectious diseases.

Some mothers who would like to breast feed their babies but do not have enough milk for the babies needs. In such cases, doctors often recommended bottle feeding the infants as well as breast feeding them. Sometimes this is done by taking turns breast feeding and bottle feeding or which is otherwise known as combined feeding.

To increase the quantity or breast milk, the mothers can take adequate calories and especially carbohydrate, green leafy vegetables, fruits and drink, plenty of fluids like milk, barley water etc. Anxiety and over work may also reduce breast milk.

Most doctors agree that there are advantages and disadvantages to breastfeeding. They also feel that the advantages outweigh the disadvantages.

Advantages of Breast Feeding

The most appropriate baby food is the mother's milk. The mother's milk has all the nutrients needed by the baby in just right proportions. This milk is safe, sterile and contains antibodies which provide immunity against diseases. The initial milk has colostrum, thick yellowish milky secretion, that has a high antibody content. It should be definitely fed to the child to provide natural immunity.

Babies who are breast fed have lesser ailments and have better nutrient formula and unsanitary conditions among the poor cause diarrhea and other gastric intestinal problems resulting in malnutrition. Frequent sucking stimulates the production of milk. Feeding the baby is satisfying both mother and child.

In the case of artificially acquired immunity the weakened on dead germs are introduced into the body and the body is stimulated to produce its own antibodies without actually having the disease. This is less painful than the naturally acquired immunity.

Disadvantages of Breast Feeding

Breast feeding may in some cases make her feel uncomfortable, tired, nervous and irritable. It keeps her more housebound than bottle feeding does.

It often leads to a temporary gain in weight. If the mother becomes emotionally disturbed, like tense, nervous or over tired, the amount and quality of her milk will be affected. Breast fed babies often become so used to being fed by one person that they have a hard time adjusting to being fed by other people when breast feeding ends.

Feeding Time

New born baby stomach can hold only about 2 tablespoon of food. So feeding should be frequent. The infant requires 2-3 ounce of breast milk per day per pound of its body weight. Mothers fed babies whenever they seemed hungry or whenever they cried, i.e., self demand schedule. Feed the baby when he is hungry and let him sleep as long as he wants to, within a few weeks he will make a schedule of waking, feeding, and sleeping which will be fairly regular. Normally the weight at birth of an well fed healthy child is doubled at the end of six months trebled at the end of a year.

Breast Feed Pattern

Before each feed the mother should wash her nipples and surrounding skin with a cotton swab which has been boiled for five minutes.

Before the commenced of a feed the mother should be comfortable and relax whether in a lying down position or sitting up in bed or in a chair. The flow of milk is affected if the mother is uncomfortable and in tense.

The mother should hold her breast between her index and middle finger lightly to help the baby get a good hold on her nipple and also to ensure that his nose is free to breath and is not smothered by the breast.

If the mother's milk is too rich she should change her diet to something less heavy. Avoidable of chesse, butter, cocoa, etc., and taking plenty of water, green leafy vegetables and fresh fruits are recommended and easily digestible.

Amount of breast milk proves insufficient. Here the child cries in between feed and fails to gain weight. In such cases every attempt should be made to increase the breast milk. If this does not succeeds the child has to be given some supplementary food.

It is important that the mother and baby should be alone during the feed. This is particularly important if it is her first baby.

Feed the bay first on one breast and let him empty it before giving him the other breast. At his next feed give him the second breast first so that one breast is well emptied at each feed. Feeding from each breast should not more than ten minutes on either side. This stimulate both sides and helps to form more milk.

Artificial Feeding

Artificial milk feed has to be restored when breast milk is really insufficient. When baby is unsatisfied with the mothers milk as cries with hunger before three hours are up is not gaining weight then the mother will have to supplement the feed with artificial feeding.

Now a days various forms of milk food are available in market:

1. *Evaporated milk*: This is cow's milk from which water has been evaporated under reduced pressure to destroy the bacteria.
2. *Condensed milk*: Just as evaporated milk but high quantity of sugar ia added.
3. *Dried milk*: cow's milk which has been rapidly dried to powder at high temperature.
4. *Skimmed milk*: Prepared similar t dried milk.
5. *Dried milk with malted cereal*: It is useful when given under medical supervision commercial milk powder are available at market.

19

Prenatal Care

The prenatal period can be considered that time of development and growth of a baby prior to birth. During this time the baby is completely dependent upon the mother for its nutritional needs. This is the most important time of an individual's life as far as nutrition is concerned. This time of rapid growth and development of the baby determines whether or not the developmental potential the child has is met, not only as a baby but, for the rest of his or her life.

During the prenatal period, important organs such as the heart, brain, spinal cord and others are forming. Without the proper levels of vitamins, minerals, and trace minerals, these organs will not develop correctly and birth defects can occur. One example of this is a condition, called spinal bifida, in which the spinal cord does not develop completely before birth. This condition is linked to low levels of vitamins B_6, B_{12} and folic acid in the mother during the prenatal period. Many physicians have realized that it is impossible for the mother to meet the vitamin and mineral needs of her baby and herself through her regular diet. Therefore, the physician recommends a prenatal vitamin in an attempt to meet those needs. However, most of the prenatal vitamins that are prescribed fall short in the form and amount of many minerals and vitamins that are needed.

The prenatal period is the most important period of time for the physical development of a human being.

Many of the problems seen today during the prenatal period can be avoided, both for the mother and the baby. Supplementation is necessary due to the inadequate amounts of mineral and vitamins in our modern food supply. Even by eating a "perfect" diet, which is almost impossible for the average woman to do, several nutrients would not be present in high enough quantities to avoid these problems.

Prenatal development is divided into three trimesters. During the first two months the developing human is referred to as an embryo. The embryo has three layers from which all body organs develop. During the second trimester the developing human is referred to as a fetus. During the third trimester, the individual is a baby which if born prematurely could survive with extra support. Premature births prior to the third trimester are less likely to survive, even with extraordinary medical care in a neonatal intensive care unit.

Sign

- Tender, swollen breasts
- Fatigue
- Implantation bleeding
- Nausea or vomiting
- Increased sensitivity to odours
- Food aversions
- Frequent urination
- A missed period
- Your basal body temperature stays high
- The proof: A positive home pregnancy test.

Pregnancy Disorders

During pregnancy, women may develop disorders that are not directly related to pregnancy. Some disorders increase the risk of problems for pregnant women or the fetus. They include disorders that cause a high fever, infections, and disorders that require abdominal surgery. Certain disorders are more likely to occur during pregnancy because of the many changes pregnancy causes in a woman's body. Examples are thromboembolic disease, anemia, and urinary tract infections.

Pregnancy Complications

Pregnancy complications are problems that occur only during pregnancy. They may affect the woman, the fetus, or both and may occur at different times during the pregnancy. For example, complications such as a dislocated placenta (placenta previa) or premature detachment of the placenta from the uterus (placental abruption) can cause bleeding from the vagina during the last 3 months of pregnancy. Women who bleed at this time are at risk of losing the baby or of bleeding excessively (hemorrhaging) or dying during labour and delivery. However, most pregnancy complications can be effectively treated.

Pregnancy Hazards

The fetus is not immune from the outside world. In fact, some things can be damaging to the unborn child. These are called teratogens, and often result in birth defects. They include such things as maternal disease, poor nutrition, stress, pollutants, and cigarette smoking. Some of the most troubling teratogens are alcohol and drugs.

It is critical to the development of the fetus that expectant mothers avoid teratogens, and receive good prenatal care. Other prenatal hazards involve genetic birth defects.

Care of Pregnant Lady

A major part in a baby's development is directly linked to the mother. To ensure that the baby stays healthy and continues normal development, you may have to make some changes. Pregnant women are encouraged not to use drugs, alcohol, or nicotine as this can seriously affect the baby's development. As a mother you should avoid drinking caffeinated beverages such as coffee and soda while increasing water consumption. Though this all may seem difficult, you are taking an active part in keeping your baby healthy.

Exercising is also very important when pregnant. Although, while exercising, there are many warnings you must heed to prevent any injury to either you or your child.

Some tips on what you should avoid in exercising while pregnant:

- Don't begin a workout without a warm up
- Don't exercise flat on your back, it can decrease the blood flow to your uterus
- Don't get dehydrated or overheated
- Don't get too fatigued

Some Safe Sports to Pursue During Pregnancy:

- Walking a 12-15 minute mile
- Swimming, because you are using your arms and legs, but the water is supporting your weight is a great exercise to do while pregnant
- Tennis is acceptable, but balance may be a problem
- Golf and bowling are also good recreational exercises, but they do nothing to condition the heart. In these, as in tennis, you may find you have some difficulty in keeping your balance.

20

The Intra-Natal Care

The word Infant derives from the Latin in-fans, meaning unable to speak. It is commonly used as a slightly more formal word for baby (the youngest category of child). A newborn infant is known as a neonate (neonatal) after the final stage of gestation. Mothers milk is the only source of every thing required for the new born baby except air. The neonate is constantly and rapidly changing, both structurally and physiologically. In the uterus, the fetus is living in a warm, moist, protected environment, and receiving all its needs from the mother. Major metabolic and physiological changes occur in the transition from a fetus to the newborn.

Meaning of Intra-natal Period

The care which is given at the time of birth is known as intra-natal care. The term neonate means new born. This term suggests complete helplessness. Although the time needed to bring about the adjustments in locate from the mother's body to the world outside requires at least 2 weeks. The period of the partunate refers to the time when the birth process is actually taking place and the period of the neonate means new born. The period of partunate covers the first 25 or 33 minutes after birth. The care which can be taken in this period is cutting of the umbilical cord, separating the infant and the infant becomes distinct and independent individual.

Adjustment After Birth

After living in the mother's body for about nine months, baby go through quite a change at birth. Adjusting to life outside the mother is a challenge for them. It takes a week or two after birth for babies to adjust to their new world.

There is birth trauma or psychological shock that results when the new born baby separated from the mother.

Before birth, oxygen comes from the placenta through the umbilical cord. When the cord is cut after birth, the infant must inhale and exhale air. The birth cry normally comes when breathing begins and thus serves to inflate the lungs.

Helplessness

The new born baby are helplessness. This is due to the undeveloped state of the body and nervous system. There are five important areas in which this lack of development plays an important role in contributing to the helplessness of the new born. They are:

1. Inability to maintain homeostasis.
2. Inability to control motor activity.
3. Inability to communicate.
4. Undeveloped state of sense organs.
5. State of daze.

Physiological Changes of New Born Baby

At birth, most neonates:

- the limited fat stores which are present are not readily available for metabolism
- limited glycogen stores rapidly after birth
- poor gluconeogenic capacity (synthesis of glucose by the liver)

- neonate have low iron stores
- immature intestines
- immature digestive capabilities,
- low activities of all pancreatic enzymes
- low activities of stomach pepsin
- low activities of many intestinal enzymes
- immature stomach acid generating capacity
- high rennin activity–for precipitation of casein, curd formation in the stomach
- increasing lactase activity–for breakdown of lactose in the intestine
- high salivary lipase activity–for breakdown of milk triglycerides

Normal New Born Weights and Measurements

After birth the baby's weight and measurements is about:

- weight: 7-8 lbs
- length: 19-21 inches
- vision: 20/40–vision is clear at a 12 inch distance

Within the first five minutes after birth the infant is assessed for his or her general health according to the Apgar scale:

- Evaluations
- heart rate
- respiratory effort
- muscle tone
- body colour

Development of New Born Baby

1. The largest and most important neuro development in the early stages of the life of the fetus

include the basic structure of the brain, the development of the nerve tracks, the development of the sensory organs, and the basic connections and pathways. These all occur purely by the genetic encoding of the cells in the central nervous system and the genetically driven biochemical processes that guide it.

2. In the second stage of development, the basic structure of the eyes and ears with their pathways into central nuclei and then to the cortex is genetically-driven. The visual and auditory cortex areas will develop in anticipation of need and without stimulation. However, how they develop and what they are capable of responding to in later life is influenced by the stimuli that they receive during certain periods of their development. These sensory organs are genetically developed but environmentally modified.

3. In the third stage of development, the processes are almost entirely driven by responses to stimulation or use of the environment of the architectural setting, even though the process was originally structured by genetics. New pathways, memory circuits, and the whole range of new connections for the neurons in the cortex of the brain are made in response to stimuli.

Care

As soon as the baby is born, wipe the babies mouth , nose face and body with a piece of clean cloth, but never with cotton or paper tissues. Move him carefully to a clean spot, cover the body with clean cloth or blanket. But leave his head uncovered for breathing. The umbilical cord should be tied lightly in two places about 2 inches apart wit a clean piece twine. Lay the baby in a warm and comfortable place.

21

Sex Development

Sexual health is more than the absence of sexual pathology. The anatomy, gender and function of the human body is the foundation of identity. The awareness of the sexual self as an integrated aspect of identity begins in infancy with the attitudes about the physical body communicated by the caretakers.

The life instinct have as their goal the preservation of life and the preservation of the species. The best known and most minutely analyzed group of life instinct are the sexual instincts. The general characteristics of the sexual instincts area as follows, they are numerous arising from many bodily sources. In the early stages of development the serve the aim of self preservation, from which they gradually detach themselves and acquire their own the own aims. The sexual instincts do not appear suddenly at puberty but go through a course of development beginning at in early infancy.

Stages of Sexual Development

Sigmund Freud (1856-1939) is probably the most well known theorist when it comes to the development of personality. *Freud's Stages of Psychosexual Development* are, like other stage theories, completed in a predetermined sequence and can result in either successful completion or a healthy personality or can result in failure, leading to an unhealthy personality. This theory is probably the most well known as well as the most controversial, as Freud believed that we develop through stages based upon a particular erogenous zone. During each stage, an unsuccessful completion means that a child becomes fixated on that particular erogenous zone and either over or under-indulges once he or she becomes an adult.

1. Oral Stage *(Birth to 18 Months)*: During the oral stage, the child if focused on oral pleasures (sucking). Too much or too little gratification can result in an Oral Fixation or Oral Personality which is evidenced by a preoccupation with oral activities. This type of personality may have a stronger tendency to smoke, drink alcohol, over eat, or bite his or her nails. Personality wise, these individuals may become overly dependent upon others, gullible, and perpetual followers. On the other hand, they may also fight these urges and develop pessimism and aggression toward others.

2. Anal Stage *(18 Months to Three Years)*: The child's focus of pleasure in this stage is on eliminating and retaining feces. Through society's pressure, mainly via parents, the child has to learn to control anal stimulation. In terms of personality, after effects of an anal fixation during this stage can result in an obsession with cleanliness, perfection, and control (anal retentive). On the opposite end of the spectrum, they may become messy and disorganized (anal expulsive).

3. Phallic Stage *(Ages Three to Six):* The pleasure zone switches to the genitals. Freud believed that during this stage boy develop unconscious sexual desires for their mother. Because of this, he becomes rivals with his father and sees him as competition for the mother's affection. During this time, boys also develop a fear that their father will punish them for these feelings, such as by castrating them. This group of feelings is known as Oedipus Complex. Later it was added that girls go through a similar situation, developing unconscious sexual attraction to their father.

According to Freud, out of fear of castration and due to the strong competition of his father, boys eventually decide to identify with him rather than fight him. By identifying with his father, the boy develops masculine characteristics and identifies himself as a male, and represses his sexual feelings toward his mother. A fixation at this stage could result in sexual deviancies (both overindulging and avoidance) and weak or confused sexual identity according to psychoanalysts.

4. Latency Stage *(Age Six to Puberty)*: It's during this stage that sexual urges remain repressed and children interact and play mostly with same sex peers.

5. Genital Stage *(Puberty on)*: The final stage of psychosexual development begins at the start of puberty when sexual urges are once again awakened. Through the lessons learned during the previous stages, adolescents direct their sexual urges onto opposite sex peers, with the primary focus of pleasure is the genitals.

Sigmund Freud's Theory is quite complex and although his writings on psychosexual development set the groundwork for how our personalities developed, it was only one of five parts to his overall theory of personality. He also believed that different driving forces develop during these stages which play an important role in how we interact with the world.

Sexual Health

It would appear that human sexual expression follows a logical, orderly and self regulating developmental pattern in much the same way as other aspects of human behaviour and that psychosexual disorders may be the result of the interruptions of that sequential growth process. It is well to remember that prior to the Victorian idealization of childhood innocence, children were commonly used and abused physically and psychologically.

The development and expression of the erotic response throughout the human lifespan is not a well studied phenomenon, and normative data have not been compiled for sexual behaviours of childhood and adolescence. As we know it, the erotic response consists of a complex interplay of physiological and psychological factors that are highly susceptible to familial, religious and cultural folkways, mores and attitudes. The styles of acceptable sexual attitude and expression fluctuate historically and culturally between generally positive and generally negative polarities.

The impacts of this often unconscious attitude on child rearing are the overt and/or covert discouragement of sexual interest, curiosity, expression and sexual behaviour of children in the presence of adults.

Sexually *permissive* cultures not only allow a less fettered expression of adult sexuality, but may give little attention to the sexual behaviours of children as long as they are not blatantly displayed.

Sexually *supportive* cultures, believing that sex is indispensable to human happiness, encourage early sexual expression as a means of developing adult sexual competency and positive sexual attitudes. The children in sexually permissive and sexually supportive societies display a similar developmental pattern that is not apparent in sexually *restrictive* and sexually *repressive* societies:

Infancy, there is usually manual and oral genital stimulation of children of both sexes by parents as a means of comforting and pacifying them (most frequently between mothers and sons).

Early Childhood, masturbation alone and in

groups, leads to exploration and experimentation among children of same and opposite gender.

Late Childhood (prepubescent) is characterized by heterosexual role modelling and attempted intercourse (girls may begin having regular coitus with older boys).

Pubescence, girls rapidly accelerate into a phase of intense sexual experience, culminating in the acquisition of basic sexual techniques at the adult level. Boys follow a similar pattern, but their learning process is not as rapid or complete because they are usually experimenting with younger girls. Heterosexual patterns replace masturbation and homosexual activities for the majority of both boys and girls.

Adolescence, there is increased sexual activity with peers and adults for both boys and girls; and it is believed that birth control is facilitated by the practice of multiple partners. Marriage is common for late adolescent girls, but boys may delay marriage for economic considerations and continue their adolescent sex patterns for longer.

Sex Education

Sex is a lot more then just how babies are, made. It includes the whole subjects of how men and women get along with each other and what their respective places in the world are.

Sex education is not just a lecture at school level or a talk by a parents at home. Whatever be the way, a child is learning about the facts of life al through his childhood. A child begins his sex education as soon as he can sense how is mother and father get along with each other in general and how they feel about their children. The curiosity stage from 2-3 years is the time when a child begins to get more exact ideas about the things that are connected with sex.

At school, could help much, having ad discussing pets. Facts can thus be leant in an impersonal situation. Biology classes could include simple discussion on reproduction etc.

At puberty it is very important the parents discuss with the children about the changes about to occur.

Sex education involves not mere information but an attempt be made to establish a healthy attitude. This is possible only when spontaneous questions asked by the children be answered as truthfully as possible and with no suggestion of shame or of there being something essentially disgraceful and wrong about sex.

22

Play Development

Play is one of the most powerful vehicles children have for trying out and mastering new skills, concepts, and experiences. Play can help children develop the knowledge they need to connect in meaningful ways to the challenges they encounter in school. Play also contributes to how children view themselves as learners. As they play, they resolve confusing social, emotional, and intellectual issues by coming up with new solutions and ideas. They experience the sense of power that comes from being in control and figuring things out on their own (something children often do not get to do in real life). This helps them develop a positive attitude toward learning.

Do a lot of to help child develop play that supports her social, emotional, and intellectual development. Here are some suggestions:

- Encourage and value play that is appropriate to the age and individual interests and needs of child.
- Help child bring his own experiences into his play. Children's play is usually more creative and less imitative when it grows out of their daily lives. For instance, providing empty food cartons and a simple toy cash register after a trip to the supermarket can help child start recreating his experience through play.
- Watch child as she plays to see what she is working on and what interests her. This can help provide

ideas about what play materials and other input might further develop her play.

- Choose new toys carefully. Toys that can be used in many ways usually promote the most valuable play. They give children many opportunities to invent new uses for them over time. Too many toys, or a constant barrage of new ones, can prevent children from doing this.
- Find ways to interact regularly (but not always) with your child as she plays. Getting involved with kids as they play — as long as you're not interrupting or taking over — shows them that adults value play.
- Try to have regular, uninterrupted playtime in child's life. This tells him that play is important. It also helps him develop the skills he needs over time to become involved in meaningful and satisfying play. For children who are heavily dependent on television, develop this routine gradually and help children figure out how to begin their play.
- Work to counteract the gender, racial, and cultural stereotypes and violence that characterize many toys. Stereotypes limit children from developing their full potential. Children sort out who they and other people are through their play. Keep this in mind when choosing new toys and try openly talking with child about these issues when they come up.
- When child does engage in violent, imitative play based on TV shows, movies or toys, help her bring in her own creativity and imagination. However you view this kind of play, the more you can help your child's play become creative, the less violent it will be.
- Make thoughtful choices about the role of media in your child's life. What and how much children see in the media can have an enormous impact on their play. TV takes time away from play activities and media content greatly influences play. So, try to develop

rules-for example, about screen time and screen content.

Types of Play

Knowing the types of play for a toy is essential to mother as they assess the environment in which the child is learning, the specific interests of the child, or the areas in which the child needs development.

1. *Active Play:* Play that involves movement and physical activity. Active play is the perfect type of play to tucker any youngster out! Whether running around in the yard, or building sand castles at a local playground, active play is an essential part of a child's development. Some examples of active play are: Riding Bikes Swinging at the playground Kickball.
2. *Cooperative Play:* Play for your child and a group of friends. Cooperative play can take place almost anywhere — outside on the playground or downstairs in the basement. In any environment, children learn from watching other children play and interacting with them socially. Some fun cooperative play activities are: Interactive pretend play Basketball Board games Game time, make believe time — it's all fun time when other children are around to take part in play!
3. *Creative Play:* Play that explores your child's imagination and makes something out of nothing! A box of crayons, construction paper, pipe cleaners, scissors and glue. They are all staples in the home, but when they come together in the hands of a child, they become magical works of art. But, creativity extends beyond art, entering a world of music, dance, building — even dirt! Creative play includes such things as: Painting sculpting play dough building or creating crafts. Providing a child a creative outlet will lead to

many amazing things, and as you may know already, some not so amazing things if it involves drawing on furniture or a wall!

4. *Dramatic Play:* Play that involves pretend and make believe, or whatever the imagination dreams. Have you ever found a child in your clothes? Carrying your briefcase? Wearing your old uniform? What seems commonplace to you opens a whole new world of possibilities to a child. Dramatic play can include: Simple role playing Using props to create a "new" environment creating scenes or situations with dolls and puppets. Children love role-playing and exploring worlds outside of their everyday, creating new and fun situations with every costume and prop. Imagine what they think you do at work!
5. *Manipulative Play:* Play that involves hand-eye coordination and motor skills. Children need the opportunity to work on finer skills that involve a little more control and direction. Manipulative play develops the sense of coordination, challenging their little fingers to follow the lines or use their tools properly. Some examples of manipulative play are: Colouring, especially in a defined area paper crafts and art involving moving parts that need to be "put together". Using a safe and simple tool kit to help with tasks around the house. Cutting out a sunshine for the window or painting within the lines — all these activities are the perfect exercise for this type of play.
6. *Quiet Play:* Play that keeps children's mouths shut but their minds open. Playtime for children should have the opportunity to be quiet — the playtime for which adults are sometimes grateful! Children need quiet time to intently digest the items in their learning environment, like books

and puzzles. Quiet play provides children an opportunity to think and reason and can include such activities as: Beading a necklace working on puzzles reading or looking at pictures. By providing a silent environment, children can focus on their toys and playthings and really get down to the work of being a child. After all, play is the work of children!

7. *Motor/Physical Play:* Motor play provides critical opportunities for children to develop both individual gross and fine muscle strength and an overall integration of muscles, nerves, and brain functions. Recent research has confirmed the critical link between stimulating activity and brain development. Young children must have ample opportunities to develop physically, and motor play instills this disposition toward physical activity in young children.
8. *Social Play:* A variety of opportunities for children to engage in social play are the best mechanisms for progressing through the different social stages. By interacting with others in play settings, children learn social rules such as, give and take, reciprocity, cooperation, and sharing. Through a range of interactions with children at different social stages, children also learn to use moral reasoning to develop a mature sense of values. To be prepared to function effectively in the adult world, children need to participate in lots of social
9. *Constructive Play:* Constructive play is when children manipulate their environment to create things. This type of play occurs when children build towers and cities with blocks, play in the sand, construct contraptions on the woodworking bench, and draw murals with chalk on the sidewalk. Constructive play allows children to

experiment with objects; find out combinations that work and don't work; and learn basic knowledge about stacking, building, drawing, making music and constructing. It also gives children a sense of accomplishment and empowers them with control of their environment. Children who are comfortable manipulating objects and materials also become good at manipulating words, ideas and concepts.

10. *Fantasy Play:* Children learn to abstract, to try out new roles and possible situations, and to experiment with language and emotions with fantasy play. In addition, children develop flexible thinking; learn to create beyond the here and now; stretch their imaginations, use new words and word combinations in a risk-free environment, and use numbers and words to express ideas, concepts, dreams, and histories. In an ever-more technological society, lots of practice with all forms of abstraction - time, place, amount, symbols, words, and ideas - is essential.

23

Baby Care

Parents are responsible for the proper up bringing of their children child rearing calls for a lot of attention, time energy money and commitment that goes with parenthood. The role of mother is very vital in up bringing of here child very often the mother will need the help and support of her husband, parents in laws and other family members in bringing up the children. The help may also be hired from other sources.

The upbringing of children is a real challenge when both parents are working urbanization desire to be independent and breakdown of joint families force the working patents to leave their small infants/children under the care and supervision of parent substitutes.

Needs of Infants and Small Children

The parents look forward to have their own children to lone and to cherish. Having a child at home means that one should be prepared for all basic needs of the baby every child needs to:

- Pre-loved and feel physically mentally, and socially secure.
- Have food for optimum growth and development
- Be clothed for protection against all possible weather conditions. Clothes also contribute to one's personality in any social set up.
- Have a shelter/home that will provide protection against natural calamities. Shelter

also provides the much needed physical security against thieves burghers and bad elements.

- Sleep soundly, peaceful sleep increases anabolic activities that promote growth among infants and children.
- Be toilet trained in due course. It develops good hygienic habits among children.
- Exercise for the proper tuning up of muscles. Physical fitness is important for each child. A healthy child is capable of having a lot of physical strength that can be learning among children.
- Develop good behaviour needed for proper socializations. Children learn social values and desirable social behaviour from family school and social environment. Parents and siblings are same of the first role models in the life of a child.
- Have control over their emotions small children grow up to be emotive secure and stable when they have a laving and a supportive family.
- Name proper medical care, protection against childhood diseases promotes good health. Each child needs to be immunized to acquire resistance against diseases.
- Be educated, reading, writing and arithmetic are essential in day-to-day life. Parents provide toys and baby to books to promote the hearing skills among their loved ones. A home is an essential preparatory schools in the life of each child. The parents should teach the children only when they are ready to learn.

What is Substitute Child Care?

You are man familiar with the needs of small

children. These are generally fulfilled by parents in the family. Economic factors often force the mothers to take up jobs. Consequently need to young ones be taken care of by olden siblings, neighbours, or relativeness etc. What role are the siblings, relatives and neighbour playing in bringing up the children? They are mother substitutes while she is at work.

Hence substitute child care can be defined as the care rendered to the child to meet the basic needs in the absence of mother/parent". Substitute cause can be made available both at home (siblings, relatives) and outside (crèche/day care centers).

Kind of Substitute Child Care

Substitute child care is provided by the following:

(a) Older siblings

(b) Reatives/neighbours.

(c) Hired help

(d) Crèche/day care centers

(e) Vice-nursery/nursery school Balwadi

Siblings Care is very common among families in low income group. Infants and children are left under the care of a slightly older child. You might find a 6 years old child looking after two to three smaller siblings, Slightly older children are not mature enough to care for the young ones. Hence it might be better idea to find an alternative get safe substitute child care centre.

Relations and Neighbors can and do play important role in the up bringing of small children in the home itself. Presence of elders in a family with children is a big boom. Grand parents in a family provide very lowing and safe child care. Neighbours can be a family away from your own family. In the absence of suitable mother substitute neighbours can provide much needed substitute child care. This sort of child care is generally of a short duration.

Hired help is a common features in affluent under families. One should carefully interview the hired help (Ayah/maid servant) as regards their reliability and experience of being able to provide for all the basic needs of the young one.

Care of the Baby

Mother of the baby often wants very much to take care of her own child but is persuaded to let someone else more experienced do this for her.

The most of obvious thing about the behaviour of any new born infant is his complete helplessness.

When a need arises his only means of tension reduction is random motor discharge. Unable to move about, to keep warm, to feed, to avoid danger, the infant is entirely dependent on his mother or some other person who takes her place.

No two babies are exactly alike and every mother has to find out how to apply what she has been taught meet the needs of her own particular child. A little baby should not be startled unnecessarily when pick him up more slowly, putting your hand under his back as you lift him so that his back, neck and head are supported. The baby should never be picked up by his arms.

The average infant is in continuous contact with his mother. Fed fonded talked to changed, cried about, express a few of these forms of contacts. This contact is a constant sources of stimulation. The infant is encouraged to babble to form words, to move about, and eventually to sit up, to stand up and to walk.

Many mothers are afraid that they will not understand what this babies are trying to say when cry. Soon the baby will have several different cries and the mother will learn to know what each one means. The baby will cry to let the mother know when he is hungry, sleepy, uncomfortable, lonely and in pain. Then proper care is given to the child if these needs are fulfilled. The child needs care for normal and healthy growth. Child care has developed into a highly systematised since within the past hundred years. The basic needs of a child for its healthy growth and development are food, clothing and baths, fresh air, play and sleep.

Daily Care

Bath: It is most important to give the baby a bath before its 10 am feed. Do not give birth after his feed. Give orange juice before bath it will keep him from getting hungry. Water should be warm and use mild soap and soft towel. oil massage can be had before and after bath. Use power after bath to absorb moisture. Protect the naval portion

Sleep: Most babies in initial months sleep from feeding to feeding, if they are getting enough to eat and not having indigestion. There are few babies who are wakeful from the beginning. With growing with his age baby sleep less. Each baby develop his own pattern. A child by the age of two is a much more complicated being. Excitement, worries, fear of bad dreams, competition with friends and siblings may keep from getting the sleep he needs. Regarding posture of sleep the baby can his own posture of sleep.

Toilet Training: Parents make a great fuss about toilet training, work very hard on it and end up with a badly untrained child. Efforts by parents at toilet training is not required. The child gradually gains control over of his bowels and bladder as he grows.

The most that parents can do guide them a little. The best time to start any sort of training is when the baby is around 7-9 months old. If the mother is too insistent, the child may rebel, and may hold back his bowel, and even come to hate the potty chair or toilet seat. More care is required in the case of a constipated child. The pan associated with the bowel movement is transferred to the potty chair. The child just does not dare let it come out at any time. This causes a viscous circle because the longer the movement stays in, the harder it gets. It is wise to leave the bowel training entirely up to the child.

Urine Training: The child has learnt to become dry in the daytime by the time he is 1-2 years old. The mother can only show where to urinate but cannot train or time urination. The child learns to control his bladder for longer time as he grows up. He can now hold on and let go and wants to perform like others in the household. The mother should not start any sort of training till the baby has learnt to be dry for at least two hours. Then she can lead him when the bladder id full, so that he does not know what is expected of him and that too pretty soon. This is usually when he is 12-15 months. Accidents can happen when he is excited, unhappy, resentful, ill. But the mother should not make an issue of it, and treat it.

24

Growth and Development

Developmental psychology studied all the changes in physical, mental, and social functioning that occur through out the life span from conception to death. Development refers to the process of change in growth and capability over time as a function of both maturation and interaction with the environment. The constant interaction with the environment results in the growth and development of the innate capacities, abilities and potentialities of the child. The function of formal, informal and non-formal education is to help the child in his path of growth and development. Therefore it is imperative that the individuals supposed to be connected with the task of helping the child to grow and develop satisfactorily, must be acquainted with the nature of growth and development. It is only with a knowledge of growth and development of the learner at each stage of his life that it is possible for the teacher to guide properly, arrange the learning situations and plan the instructional programme for bringing about desirable harmonious development in their personalities. Therefore human growth and development has been accepted as one of the important study.

Meaning of Growth and Development

Most of us use the two terms growth and development interchangeably and accept them as synonymous terms. Both these terms relate to the measurement of changes occurred in the individual after conception in the womb of the mother. Change is made as the law of nature. An individual starting from a fertilized egg, turns into a full fledged human adult. In this process a cycle of change brought about by the process of growth and development in various dimensions— physical, mental, social, emotional etc. Therefore in the wider sense, both the terms growth and development can be used for any change brought about by maturation and learning and essentially is the product of both heredity and environment.

Meaning of Growth

The term is purely used as physical sense. It generally refers to an increase in size, length, height and weight, changes in the quantitative aspects come into the domain of growth.

Growth is the one of the part of developmental process. In pure sense development in its quantitative aspects is termed as growth.

Growth may be referred to describe the changes which take place in particular aspects of the body and behaviours of an organism.

Growth does not continue through out life. It stops when maturity attained.

The changes produce by growth are the subject of measurement. They may be quantified and the observable in nature.

Meaning of Development

Development by contrast refers to quantitative and qualitative changes. It may be defined as a progressive series of orderly coherent changes. Development defined as a the series of changes which an organism undergoes in passing from an embryonic state of maturity. These changes refers to physical, emotional, intellectual changes.

Development is also possible without growth as we see in the cases of some children that they do not gain in terms of height, weight or size but they do experience functional improvement or development in physical, social, emotional or intellectual aspect.

Development as said implies improvement in functioning and behaviour and hence brings quantitative changes which are difficult to be measure directly. They are assessed through keen observation in behavioural situation.

Development is a continuous process. It goes from womb to womb. It does not end with the attainment of maturity changes however small they may be, continue through out life span of an individual.

Development describe the changes in the organism as a whole and does not list the changes in parts.

Development is wider and comprehensive term. It refers to overall changes in the individual, growth is one of its part.

Significance of Developmental Changes

Developmental changes are continuous and gradual. The importance of these continuous changes among children has been highlighted by research in the field of child psychology and child education. Because of these developmental changes certain characteristics emerge in the life of an individual, which put a permanent stamps on his whole life. It is the real period of learning. In this period the most significant patterns of thought and behaviour are formed. Therefore the study of early infancy and childhood in human development is the most significant.

Stages of Growth and Development

Life begins at the moment of conception. When the ovum is fertilized by the sperm. There are certain common developmental or practical characteristics belonging to each stage. The human organism shows peculiar quantitative and qualitative changes in his body and behaviour with the help of which we can say at what particular age an individual belongs to which definite stages of his life. The span of an individual can be divided into the following stages.

Stages	*Period of approximate age*
1. Pre-natal stage	From conception to birth.
2. Infancy stage	From birth to five years.
3. Childhood stage	From 6th to 12 years or in strict sense up to the on set of puberty.
4. Adolescent stage	From the on set of puberty to the age of maturity, generally from 13 to 19 years.
5. Adulthood stage	From 20 yeas and beyond or in strict sense from the age of attaining maturity till death.

Principles of Growth and Development

Psychologists believe that an accurate picture of the principles of growth and development is essential for the teacher. They are as follows:

1. Development is a life long process.
2. Development involves change.
3. Early development is more critical than later development.

4. From infancy to childhood each individual has his own rate of growth.

5. Growth pattern is continuous and gradual.

6. Growth is a process of both differentiation and integration.

7. The effect of training varies with the stage of maturation.

8. There are wide individual difference in growth pattern.

Influence of Heredity and Environment on Growth and Development

We all have similar beginning, it is interesting to ask what makes us al so different as we grow older. One answer is that except inn the case of identical twins, we have different heredity. Another answer is that we have different environments. There is further more a constant interplay between heredity and environmental influences and our physical and mental characteristics are the complex results of both factors.

Educational Implication of Growth and Development

Knowledge of various characteristics features of child development through infancy, childhood and adolescence in indispensable for teacher owing mainly to the following reasons:

1. It gives him the most authentic knowledge regarding the human stuff that he deals with the children.

2. It enables him to understand the root causes of their good and bad behaviours of child.

3. It helps him to match his teaching, techniques, and standards to the developmental level that a child

has actually attained. He is thus enabled to avoid being too difficult, too easy or too common place in the class room.

4. By enabling him to understand his own infancy and childhood periods it facilities for him an understanding of his own self. This self understanding proves immensely helpful for him in becoming a better person and a better teacher.

25

Immunization for the Baby

Definition

Immunity can be defined as the ability of an individual to resist disease and death.

How Immunity Developed

Microorganisms and the pathogens are recognized as enemies. They contain antigens that stimulate the production of antibodies to build up body defense mechanism. The body needs to produce different antibodies for providing protection against the various disease germs.

Types

Immunity are two types, i.e., natural and acquired. Acquired immunity can be naturally ore artificially induced.

Natural immunity is present at birth. Some antibodies also get transferred from mother to the infant during breast feeding. Hence breast feeding of infants is very important.

Childhood Diseases Preventable by Immunization

Disease against which the children can be immunized?

Tuberculosis, peretusis, polio diphtheria, mumps, whooping cough tetanus, measles, hepatitis.

Immunization can be defined as “the process of developing immune bodies antibodies in an individual by artificially introducing controlled number of germs into the body. This stimulates the production of antibodies and provides immunity against diseases”.

Immunization Schedule

BCG (Bacillus Calmetle Guein)

It is named after the French bacterilogits calmetle and Guerin. It provides protectively against tuberculosis. The vaccine injected with the dermis of aim left side. It is given at birth as soon after local reaction ray occur 3-4 weeks taken.

DPT (Diphtheria, Pertussis, Tetanus)

It is a triple vaccine providing immunity against diphtheria, pertusis (whooping cough) and tetanus. The first dose is injected at the age of 6 weeks of age the subsequent two does are given at an interval of 4 weeks.

DTap is the updated version of DPT. The ‘a’ stands for “accellulan” as only a part of the pertusis bacteria is used in the vaccine.

Polio: It is an local vaccine providing immunity against attack of the crippling polio disease. It is now available in overall form and is given three doses standing at birth. The second and third doses are given at an interval of 4-8 weeks each. Additional polio vaccine doses are given to children to eradicate this disease.

MMR (Measles, Mumps and Rubella)

It is the latest vaccine providing immunity for three disease. It is given in a single dose in an injectable form at the age of 9 months. It provides immunity again mumps, measles and rubella.

Typhoid: It is a food and water borne disease caused bacillus bacteria. The disease is characterized by fever and malice. The available heat phenol inactivated typhoid vaccine provides limited protection only. It is an injectable vaccine and can be given at 2 years of age second dose can be repeated an interval of 3-6 weeks.

Hepatitis B Vaccine: It provides protection against a virus that causes inflammatic of linear resulting in jaundice. The virus is transmitted through contaminated needle and blood transfusion. New born babies are likely to get it from caring mother. It is a serious disease. First dose can be given at birth, second after 1-2 months and third 6-18 months.

(i) All vaccines should be give to the child and a prior record of these shots should be kept.

(ii) Booster doses of DPT and polio are given between 16-24 months. These are repeated when the child joins school. Tetanus is shout

lived. The tetanus shot needs to be repeated as and when the child gets an opened wound with rusted and dirty objects.

(iii) Under the national immunization programmed the children are also being given prophylactic doses of oral Vitamin A to provide protection against blindness.

Chicken Pox: Their disease is common among children and is caused by a virus. The incubation period spans 14-21 days. It .4 an air borne infection and spreads by direct and indirect contact. Coughing and sneezing by sick child release large number of germs. Sick has fever and headache. Rashes appear all over the body and cashes fill with us to form blisters and causes uncomfortable inning. Application of calamine lotion relieves itchy. The rash dries to form scabs that are infections. There is possibility of respiratory problems like pneumonia. The disease lasts for about 21 days.

Cholera: It is caused by bacillus bacteria called "vibrio-coma". It spreads fat with the consumption of infected food and mocker. The incubation period is short, i.e., 1-5 days. The disease characterized by loose watery motions that look like "rice water". It is accompanied by vomiting resulting in extreme fluid and electrolyte loss. The patient gets cramped and feels extremely thirsty. Suppression of urine leads to the accumulation of toxic materials in the body. The child should be given plenty of fluids to avoid dehydration.

Diarrhea: It is a condition where the stomach becomes loose due to infection. The infections agents and parasite's (worms) enter the system due to poor environmental sanitation and long standard of personal hygiene.

Frequently watery stools may be accompanied by stomach. The child feels neck and thirsty. Ignorant mothers try to control diarrhea by restricting the fluid intake. The child suffers dehydration which if uncontrolled could prove fatal. Skin loses its elasticity and it controlled local dehydration solution by ORS.

Dysentery: It is caused by Entamoeba histolytic and bacillus bacteria. The incubation period is short and the child and recovers within a week. The child will have stomach pain and pass frequent stools. Sometimes the stools may be accompanied by traces of mucous and blood. This results in general means. The course of treatment and control is similar as in diarrhea.

Influenza and Common Cold: These are minor ailments causingconsiderable discomfort among little babies. Influenza is caused by a virus. The incubation period is very short and the disease spreads though air as well as close contact. It is characterized by cough, running nose, sneezing and fever. It is a good practice to core young nose/mouth while sneezing.

The child should be protected from air draughts and isolated from siblings and other children. Warm milk, soups and vegetables broths and egg-nog etc. can be given to the child build up strength to fight the disease germs. It is a good practice to cover your mouth/ nose while sneezing.

Ear Infections: Accompany cough, cold influenza and other respiratory problems. The discharge and wax accumulate in the care and cause terrible plain to the child. The child may also have fever at times immediate treatment provides relief and safety against possible hearing impairment.

Sore Eyes: These eyes are quite common among children living in slums and poor sanitary conditions. The eyes become sticky, cause itching and have burning sensations. The eyelids get swollen. It is highly communicable conditions. Eyes could be mashed and given hot fermentations with like maximum saline water.

Scabies: The baby skin is soft and tender poor personal and environmental sanitation results in scabies that is can by ichnites. The itching spread fast. The scabies can be controlled by bathing the child with antiseptic and genetic soap. The personal clothing and bedding of all family members needs to be cleaned and sunned.

Boils: Boils in baby skin have pus-forming staphylococcus bacteria. The boils are ores inflamed and painful. Clean the boils with worm saline water and apply antiseptic cream.

Thread Worm Infection: In female the worm is 8-13 long and the male warm is half the size. The warms attach themselves to the folds of skin around anus. These can be seen with naked eye at the anus and cause a lot of itching. The itching fingers and nails pick up the eggs laid by the female worm and find entry into the mouth. The eggs turn into larve into the duodenum and find entry into the mouth. The eggs turn into lavell into the duodenum and pass down to the large intestine and out to anus as worm. These worms loss of appetite, restlessness, cough, sleepiness, and even convulsion. The nails should be trained and the hands kept clean. Son child's wrappings bed cloths and towels to sleep with their siblings till cured, clean the child's anus thoroughly after the child has passed the stools. Smear anus with ammoniated inercucy ointment.

What are Immunizations?

Immunity is when antibodies fight infectious diseases and stay in your system, even after the disease is gone, to protect you from getting sick again. Newborn babies have natural immunity to many diseases because they have antibodies they got from their mothers, but this immunity wears off before the baby's first birthday. Even after the natural immunity wears off, children can be protected against many diseases by vaccinating them against those diseases.

Why Immunizations are Important

Vaccines are one of the greatest achievements of medical science and public health. But in spite of the dramatic declines in vaccine-preventable diseases, such diseases still exist, particularly in developing countries. Children need immunizations to keep them healthy and to protect them from dangerous childhood diseases. Without vaccines, epidemics of vaccine-preventable diseases would return, resulting in increased illness, disability, and death.

Unfortunately some children and adults do not get all of their necessary vaccinations. This is caused by fear, religious or personal beliefs, lack of access to health care, or a lack of understanding. There also are many misconceptions about vaccines that keep people from being properly protected. Immunizations for childhood diseases are now required by law in all states, and children may not be allowed to attend day care or school or participate in sports activities if they have not been immunized.

26

Common Problems of Childhood

Childhood Diseases

Introduction: In our developing countries nearly a quarter million children die in a week and many millions suffer from poor health and morbidity. Ignorance, as regards the protective of health among children leads to high mortality rate, child is healthy when he/she does not suffer from diseases. Freedom from diseases promotes good health, long life, faithful productive years and economic prosperity of an individual and the nation.

Health and disease differ like day and night as can be seen below:

Health can be defined as the experience of success experienced by an organism in its efforts to respond adoptively to environmental challenges.

Disease defined as the experience of failure experienced by an organism in its efforts to respond adoptively to environmental challenges.

These diseases occur frequently amongst children, list are given belong: mumps, diarrhea, measles, cholera, chicken pox, polio, whooping cough, cough and cold, diphtheria, earache, worm infestation etc.

Diseases are of two main types: they are communicable and non-commercial diseases. Communicable diseases spread rapidly through the medium of hast, air food, water, contact, insects bites and agents.

Agents, (pathogens include microorganism like bacteria, virus and worms.

Communicable disease means it spreads from one person to another.

Non-communicable disease means it does not spread from one person to another.

Prevention and Control of Communicable Diseases

Communicable diseases can be prevented and controlled by the following three factors:

Importance personal by given and sanitation has also been formally studies in your health classes.

Barriers Against Disease Germs

Body resists the entry of disease germs and after resistance in many ways.

Barriers of Body

(i) *Skin:* The given cannot find entry unless the skin in damaged. Much secreted by mucous membranes repel bacteria.

(ii) *Saliva:* The antiseptic qualities of the saliva are well known. The germ can also be expelled from the body by coughing out.

(iii) *Tear Glands:* Produce secretion containing lysozyme which has a potential of billing and washing away the germs.

(iv)*Nasal:* Opening have cillia that sweep out the germs to some extent. Sneezing can expel bacteria.

(v) *Urine and Force:* Besides excreting body waste, also gets rid of some of the pathogens.

(vi)*Stomach:* Secrets Pepsin hydrochloric acid that burns away some of the groups. The stomach has the unique ability of rejecting its contents if one has consumed highly contaminated food.

(vii) *Blood:* Contains white blood cells. The WBCs more like the single called amoeba. They engulf the bacteria and release a ferment to liquefy bacteria.

(viii) *Lymph Nodes:* These nodes engulf the disease germs and kill them. The lymph nodes may become enlarge.

Protection and Prevention Childhood Diseases

Protect Your Child

We have record or near record low levels of vaccine-preventable childhood diseases in the United States, but that does not mean these have disappeared. Many of the viruses and bacteria are still circulating in this country or are only a plane ride away. That's why it's important that children, especially infants and young children, receive recommended immunizations on time.

SECTION-C
CHILD PSYCHOLOGY

27

Child Psychology

Meaning: Child development deals with growth and development of characteristics. It is concerned with the discovery, interpreting and productively individual development. It is also concerned with child guidance and counseling children.

Child-psychology and child development deals with under finding of growth and development patterns and the development of various characteristics in children.

Child development is defined as a branch of knowledge concerned with both the nature of development and regulation of significant structural functional and behavioural changes occurring in children as they advanced in age and maturity. It deals with understanding the development of characteristics of children and the process through which development starts.

Nature: Child development is nature source psychologist observe, describe, measures and relate phenomena as they occurs naturally in unconscious situation child development based on naturalistic observation. It manipulate emotions attitudes, and value among the children concept of development free-supposes that there is a continuity in development. This continuity is lawful and is observed between successive stage of an ongoing growth process and that properties of earlier phase contributes to the properties of subsequent phase. These changes are progressive heredity and environment facilities contribute to process to change. There is also reciprocal changes between organism and the environment.

Importance: Child psychology or developmental psychology attempts to understand complex behaviour by studying their simpler beginnings. Child psychology studied the meaning of childhood, children as peoples the role of heredity in the child's development, parental influences, the relationship between physical and psychological characteristics, child training methods, intelligence, sex difference etc.

Importance of child psychology can be illustrated given the point of widen of parents, teachers and guidance experts.

Parents: It enables them to keep a record of the growth of the child of they are interested. The parents became able to know that is the critical period in development, about enriched environment, hour such facilities created, how the baby will reached, his curiosity etc.

Child psychology enable the parents to know the technical leas of dealing with childhood emotions and when resultant frustration in a more heal way than by spacing on using the road only. The apply the motivational and learning principles to bring changes on their children. Parents can guide their children according to childhood interest. They can held them to develop socialization and cognitive development. Child psychology is useful to parents in the area of language and socialization.

Teacher: Child psychology is useful to teacher in early childhood Received teacher know the basic needs of children that are to be compiled in school without which the child areas quit school. Child psychology enables teacher to be acquainted with wide stones of development. It enables teacher to find out the behaviour problems in school teacher uses most observational techniques. Many teacher spot the child because they do not know the mental state of child. The knowledge of child psychology in meaningful.

Guidance Experts: In our country child guidance has not been developed except is very big cities and that two very rarely psychologically oriented. These are medically designed with child guidance clinic.

Child guidance is necessary. For this purpose through and comprehensive understanding of child development is essential so, understanding of the child psychology is necessary because if contributes to later development of personality and behaviour.

Scope

(i) Child psychology are so many and varied.

(ii) Child psychology helping the child who suffers from chronic behaviour problems.

(iii) Child psychology becomes useful in guidance of children.

(iv) Child psychology is necessary for child's personality development.

(v) Child psychology is essential for parents for socialization.

Objectives

Child psychologist have accepted the four fold objectives: observation, prediction, guidance, and central of child behaviour and development.

(i) Child psychology helps one to observe the child behaviour.

(ii) Child psychology helps one to predict child behaviour.

(iii) Child psychology helps one to guide child

behaviour.

(iv) Child psychology helps one to control child behaviour.

Theory of Child Psychology

Child psychology includes on understanding of the child from the time of concept, the principles by which hereditary vacant are transmitted to children, prenatal case of fetus and the mother, attention paid to factors such as maternal nutritional deficiency disease, X-ray, drugs etc., and including the development of ovum, embryo and fetus.

Child psychology concerned with behaviour of neonate. It also include study of intelligence, emotion language proficiency play, creativity and cognitive development of children.

Child psychology encompassed with the prenatal, perinatal, postnatal growth and development, bitch hazards, baby care and ailments of childhood.

Child psychology is the both the qualitative and quantitative study of children's behaviour. It studies growth and development. Growth refers in size and structure. The child grows physically and mentally. Development by contrast refers to qualitative changes. It is always progressive and coherent. It refers to the forward and definite relationship of one stage of development to the other. Growth and development are inseparable, neither takes place alone. Thus child development is a much broader field than child psychology. As it is relatively recent in origin, our knowledge of the psychological phenomenon characteristics of the childhood is rather incomplete. But there is both scientific and popular confidence in the information already available about child development. The delay and lack of motivation for the study of children is attributed to the fact that children were regarded as miniature adults and it was considered unnecessary to the study them directly. Since adult are easier to study, scientists concentrated on them and assumed that what was learned could then be applied to the understanding of children. Later with the desire to improve child behaviour and child care, and throw light on problems related to child training, child psychology as a subject of study gained importance and impetus. It started as a study of specific areas of child behaviour such as emotion, play interests and activities of the preschool and school age child, and finally developed to be the study of the pattern of behaviour development of the child.

Developmental psychology is the study of changes in behavioural and mental processes through life. Each stage of development poses its own problems. Though new problems arise through out a person's life span, development is most rapid in the first few years of life. Thus infant and children are faced with major developmental problems to solve. Two main techniques used to study the course of developmental changes are longitudinal and cross-sectional methods. In the longitudinal method, people are followed through their life span. In cross-sectional method, representative groups who are at different stages in development are compared.

28

Physical Growth

Children grow, develop, and learn throughout their lives from birth and infancy to adulthood. A child's development can be measured through social, physical, and cognitive developmental milestones. If children fail to develop properly they may be unable to reach their full potential. However, health care professionals and parents can work together as partners to help children grow up healthy and strong.

Stages of Physical Development

From the start, babies want to explore their world. They are eager to move their eyes, their mouths, and their bodies toward the people and objects that comfort and interest them. They practice skills that let them not only move closer to desired objects, but also move desired objects closer to themselves. As they grow, children's determination to master child begins life as a being with little control of movement and progresses to one who can run, jump, laugh, sing, write with a pencil and control his own small and large muscles with growing confidence. This progression is physical development.

Although humans change physically throughout life, the changes which occur during the first four years are dramatic and eagerly awaited. Muscle skills development and maintaining a healthy body are especially important to future reading, writing, and math success.

There are individual differences in the area of

physical development ranging from one month to four to six months for each particular skill.

Age	*Milestones*
The first year	A baby begins learning the basics of self-movement and begins to master the skills needed for hand-to-mouth coordination and holding objects.
Birth (0-3) months	Most infants begin to: • Raise head slightly when lying on stomach. • Hold head up for a few seconds, when supported. • Hold hand in a fist. • Lift head and chest, while lying on stomach. • Use sucking, grasping, and rooting (holding tongue to the roof of the mouth) reflexes. • Touch, pull, and tug own hands with fascination. • Repeat body movements, and enjoy doing so.
Birth (0-3) months	Most infants begin to:
3-6 months	Babies are quickly becoming stronger and more agile. Most begin to: • Roll over. • Push body forward and pull body up by grabbing the edge of a crib. • Reach for and touch objects. • Reach, grasp, and put objects in mouth. • Make discoveries with objects

(for example, a rattle makes noise when it is moved).

6-9 months

"Child-proofing" becomes important as babies get more mobile. During this time most begin to:

- Crawl.
- Grasp and pull things toward self.
- Transfer objects between hands.

9-12 months

By this time, most babies can:

- Sit without support.
- Stand unaided.
- Walk with aid.
- Roll a ball.
- Throw objects.
- Pick things up with thumb and one finger.
- Drop and pick up toys.

1-2 years

Walking and self-initiated movement become easier. Most children can:

- Walk alone.
- Walk backwards.
- Pick up toys from a standing position.
- Push and pull objects.
- Seat self in a child's chair.
- Walk up and down stairs with aid.
- Move to music.
- Paint with whole arm movement.

Balance improves and eye-hand coordination becomes more

precise. Most children can:

- Put rings on a peg.
- Turn two or three pages at a time.
- Scribble.
- Turn knobs.
- Grasp and hold a small ball; can use in combination with large motor skills to throw the ball.
- Shift marker or any drawing or painting tool from hand to hand and draw strokes.

2-3 years

Children become more comfortable with motion, increasing speed, and coordination. Most begin to:

- Run forward.
- Jump in place with both feet together.
- Stand on one foot, with aid.
- Walk on tiptoe.
- Kick ball forward.

Children are able to manipulate small objects with increased control. Most can:

- String large beads.
- Turn pages one by one.
- Hold crayon with thumb and fingers instead of fist.
- Draw a circle.
- Paint with wrist action, making dots and lines.
- Roll, pound, squeeze, and pull clay.

3-4 years

Movement and balance improve. Most children can:

- Run around obstacles.

- Walk on a line.
- Balance on one foot.
- Push, pull, and steer toys.
- Ride a tricycle.
- Use a slide without help.
- Throw and catch a ball.

Children's precision of motion improves significantly. Most are able to:

- Build a tall tower of blocks.
- Drive pegs into holes.
- Draw crosses and circles.
- Manipulate clay by making balls, snakes, etc.

4-5 years

Children are now more confident, and most are able to:

- Walk backwards.
- Jump forward many times without falling.
- Jump on one foot.
- Walk up and down stairs without assistance, alternating feet.
- Turn somersaults.

Children develop skills that will help them as they enter school and begin writing. Most can:

- Use safety scissors.
- Cut on a line continuously.
- Copy squares and crosses.
- Print a few capital letters.

29

Sensory Motor Development

Motor Development

Motor means movement. The two most studied movement abilities are walking fuse of hard as tools or pretension. Both are maturation in origin, though environment can play a role in modulating the expression of the maturation potentially.

Actually we mature to walk rather than learn to walk. The following sequence of motor development leads to walking:

1. Chin up.
2. Chest up.
3. Reach and miss.
4. Sit with support.
5. Sit lap grasp object.
6. Sit alone.
7. Stand with help.
8. Stand holding objects.
9. Creep and crawl.
10. Walk when led.
11. Pull to stand.
12. Climb stairs.
13. Stand alone.
14. Walk alone.

Perhension also follows a predictable sequence in development. It start with the baby's crude movements in direction of objects. Soon the infants proceed to simple palmar grasping and gripping an object with the palm of the hand. This is followed by more precise finger and thumb dexterity until it finally progress to opposition of the thumb and finger. This sequence of change is controlled by maturation of the nervous system, arm and hands.

Most infants develop motor abilities in the same order and at approximately the same age. In this sense, most agree that these abilities are genetically pre-programmed within all infants. The environment does play a role in the development, with an enriched environment often reducing the learning time and an impoverished one doing the opposite.

The following chart delineates the development of infants in sequential order. The ages shown are averages and it is normal for these to vary by a month or two in either direction:

2 months – able to lift head up on his own

3 months – can roll over

4 months – can sit propped up without falling over

6 months – is able to sit up without support

7 months – begins to stand while holding on to things for support

9 months – can begin to walk, still using support

10 months – is able to momentarily stand on her own without support

11 months – can stand alone with more confidence

12 months – begin walking alone without support

14 months – can walk backward without support

17 months – can walk up steps with little or no support

18 months – able to manipulate objects with feet while walking, such as kicking a ball

Stages of Motor Development

Birth to One Month

By two weeks of age your baby will probably have regained most or all of the weight that he lost in his first week.

In the next few baby to look at your face, startle with loud noises, lift his head and begin to smile spontaneously. He may even begin to recognize familiar objects and sounds.

Two Months

At this age you can expect your baby to smile, laugh and make noises, lift her head and chest up while lying on her stomach, turn toward sounds and to follow you around with her eyes. Over the next few months, developmental milestones will include rolling over, bearing weight on her legs, sitting with support and holding on to a rattle.

Four Months

At this age you can expect your baby to roll over (front to back), bear weight on her legs, sit with support, hold up her head and chest and support herself on her elbows if she is on her stomach, pull to a sitting position and hold on to a rattle. Over the next few months your baby will start to imitate speech sounds, reach for objects and sit without support.

Six Months

Your baby has probably doubled her birth weight by now. At this age you can expect her to imitate speech sounds, reach for objects, roll over, and sit without support. Over the next few months she will start to stand holding on to things, pull to a stand, jabber and combine syllables, crawl and transfer things from hand to hand.

Nine Months

At this age you can expect your baby to sit alone,

pull to a stand, stand holding on to things, jabber and imitate sounds, crawl, wave bye-bye, and begin to show separation and stranger anxiety. Over the next few months your baby will start to combine syllables, say mama/dada, walk with her hands held, and bang objects together.

Your baby will now begin to explore how things work, enjoy playing peek-a-boo and pat-a-cake and being read to. It is important to give lots of praise and many opportunities for exploration. If using a pacifier, it is a good time to start restricting its use to only when your baby is in his crib, so that his interest in it will decrease.

Twelve Months

Your baby has probably tripled her birth weight. You can expect her to combine syllables, say mama/dada, walk while holding on to things, take a few steps alone, bang objects together, enjoy reading interactively, and point to pictures. Over the next few months she will start to walk well alone, say 3-6 words, understand simple commands, and begin to use a spoon or fork.

Fifteen Months

Your baby has probably tripled her birth weight. Developmental milestones you can expect her to meet include starting to combine syllables, say mama/dada, walk alone, bang objects together, enjoy reading interactively, and point to pictures. Over the next few months she will start to say 3-6 words, understand simple commands, and begin to use a spoon or fork.

This is also a time that your child will begin to explore and try and figure out how things work and will enjoy playtime. It is important to give lots of praise and many opportunities for exploration. If using a pacifier, it is a good time to start restricting its use to only when your baby is in his crib, so that his interest in it will decrease.

Most babies take two naps (length of naps are usually very variable between different children, but naps are usually 1-1 1/2 hours each) during the day at this age and are able to sleep for the majority of the night (at least 11 hours). If not, check to make sure that your baby has a good bedtime routine and has developed the proper sleep associations.

Eighteen Months

At this age you can expect your child to walk backwards, walk up steps with her hand held, kick a ball, say 10 to 25 words, name 3 body parts, turn pages of a book and stack two blocks together. Over the next few months your child will learn new words, start to throw a ball overhand, use two word combinations, and remove clothing.

He may begin to play around other children, but it will be 'parallel play.' Children at this age are very self-centered and may play alongside each other, but it will be some time before they actually start playing together. Your child will probably not want to share his things and he may be very possessive. It is important to closely supervise children that are playing together at this age and reassure them that the other child will not keep his toys. Keep a few of his favourite items separate and not available for sharing so that he feels he has some control over things.

Two Years

At this age you can expect your child to put on clothing, brush his teeth with help, stack 4-6 blocks, combine words, know over 50 words, use pronouns (I, me, you, mine), follow two step commands, know his body parts, walk up steps, kick a ball, jump up, throw a ball overhead, and his speech should be half understandable. Over the next year his speech will become more understandable, and he will be able to name pictures and colours. If using a pacifier, it is a good time to start restricting its use to only when your baby is in his crib, so that his interest in it will decrease.

Three Years

At this age your child is becoming more independent and you can expect him to dress himself and button clothes, brush his teeth with help, stack 9-10 blocks, draw circles and squares, use scissors, walk up steps by alternating his feet, jump from a step, hop, walk on his toes, pedal a tricycle, play with imaginary friends, have a very large vocabulary and use 3-4 word sentences and his speech should be 3/4 understandable. Over the next year his speech will become fully understandable.

Three Years

At this age your child is becoming more independent and you can expect him to dress himself and button clothes, brush his teeth with help, stack 9-10 blocks, draw circles and squares, use scissors, walk up steps by alternating his feet, jump from a step, hop, walk on his toes, pedal a tricycle, play with imaginary friends, have a very large vocabulary and use 3-4 word sentences and his speech should be 3/4 understandable. Over the next year his speech will become fully understandable.

Your three year old will now begin to play cooperatively with other children in small groups, share his toys and develop friendships. Playtime will include structured games and fantasy activities.

Four Years

At this age you can expect your child to dress himself, brush his teeth without help, play board and card games and follow simple rules, name 4 colours, hop, walk down stairs alternating feet, talk in 4-5 word sentences, sing songs, listen to stories, shares things spontaneously, count to 4, and his speech should be fully understandable. Over the next few years he will be able to count to ten, recognize letters of the alphabet, and be able to learn his phone number and address.

Five Years

At this age you can expect your child to dress himself, brush his teeth without help, play cooperatively with other children, play board and card games and follow the rules, name colors, hop, walk down stairs alternating feet, skip, talk in 4-5 word sentences, sing songs, listen to stories, shares things spontaneously, recognize letters of the alphabet, print letters, know his phone number and address and his speech should be fully understandable.

Movements and Phases of Motor Development

The development of a child's motor behaviour is a sequential process. This development starts with simple reflexes to the learning of postural movements, to loco motor responses, and finally, fine manipulative movements.

Four Phases of Development

Phase 1: From reflexes to rudimentary movements such as sitting, crawling, creeping, standing, and walking. Phases (stages) of development Four phases of development are usually identified.

Phase 2: Running, climbing, jumping, balancing, catching and throwing are developed. These are sometimes labeled as the fundamental skills. These fundamental skills are common to all healthy children and normally develop in the same order as all children. Phases (stages) of development four phases of development are usually identified.

Phase 3: During late childhood, more specific movement skills will appear, while the general fundamental skills become more refined and will appear more fluid and are more automatic. Phases (stages) of development four phases of development are usually identified.

Phase 4: During adolescence the specific movements develop further and can be called specialized. This process depends of the amount of practice an individual has with specific skills, which is influenced by talent, motivation and stimulation as well as success and failure.

30

Cognitive Growth

Definition

Cognitive development is the development of the thinking and organizing systems of the brain. It involves language, mental imagery, thinking, reasoning, problem solving, and memory development.

Cognitive Development in Children

A positive role in your child's cognitive development by playing with her, having conversations with her, explaining what is happening as you go through the day together, introducing her to new activities and environments, encouraging her to explore and experiment, giving her choices, reading to her, being interested in her interests, letting her know it is okay to make mistakes, and loving and being proud of her. A child's growth and development may be divided into four periods: infancy, the preschool years, the middle childhood years, and adolescence. Immediately after birth, an infant normally loses approximately 5 per cent to 10 per cent of his or her birth weight. However, by about 2 weeks of age, an infant should start to have rapid weight gain and growth.

By 4 to 6 months of age, an infant's weight should be double the birth weight. During the second half of the first year of life, growth is not as rapid. Between the ages of 1 and 2, a toddler will gain only about 5 pounds. Weight gain will remain at about 5 pounds per year between the ages of 2 and 5.

Between the ages of 2 and 10 years, a child will continue to grow at a steady pace. A final growth spurt begins with the onset of puberty, sometime between the ages of 9 and 15.

Nutrient needs correspond with these changes in rates of growth, meaning an infant needs more calories in relation to size than a preschooler or school-age child needs. Nutrient needs increase again as a child approaches adolescence.

Piaget's Theory of Cognitive Development

Probably the most cited theory in the cognitive development in children is Jean Piaget (1896-1980). As with all stage theories, *Piaget's Theory of Cognitive Development* maintains that children go through specific stages as their intellect and ability to see relationships matures. These stages are completed in a fixed order with all children, even those in other countries. The age range, however can vary from child to child.

Sensory Motor Stage: This stage occurs between the ages of birth and two years of age, as infants begin to understand the information entering their sense and their ability to interact with the world. During this stage, the child learns to manipulate objects although they fail to understand the permanency of these objects if they are not within their current sensory perception. In other words, once an object is removed from the child's view, he or she is unable to understand that the object still exists.

The major achievement during this stage is that of Object Permanency, or the ability to understand that these objects do in fact continue to exist. This includes his ability to understand that when mom leaves the room, she will eventually return, resulting in an increased sense of safety and security. Object Permanency occurs during the end of this stage and represents the child's during the end of this stage and represents the child's ability to maintain a mental image of the object (or person) without the actual perception.

Sensory Motor Period (0 - 24 Months)

Developmental Stage and Age Characteristics Behaviours

Reflexive Stage (0-2 months)	Simple reflex activity such as grasping, sucking.
Primary Circular Reactions (2-4 months)	Reflexive behaviours occur in stereo-typed repetition such as opening and closing fingers repetitively.
Secondary Circular Reactions (4-8 months)	Repetition of change actions to reproduce interesting consquences such as kicking one's feet to more a mobile suspended over the crib.
Coordination of Secondary Reactions (8-12 months)	Responses become coordinated into more complex sequences. Actions take on an "intentional" character such as the infant reaches behind a screen to obtain a hidden object.
Tertiary Circular Reactions (12-18 months)	Discovery of new ways to produce the same consequence or obtain the same goal such as the infant may pull a pillow toward him in an attempt to get a toy resting on it.
Invention of New Means Through Mental Combination (18-24 months)	Evidence of an internal representa tional system. Symbolizing the problem-solving sequence before actually responding. Deferred imitation.

The Pre-operational Period (2-7 Years)

Pre-operational Stage: The second stage begins

after Object Permanency is achieved and occurs between the ages of two to seven years of age. During this stage, the development of language occurs at a rapid pace. Children learn how to interact with their environment in a more complex manner through the use of words and images. This stage is marked by Egocentrism, or the child's belief that everyone sees the world the same way that she does. The fail to understand the differences in perception and believe that inanimate objects have the same perceptions they do, such as seeing things, feeling, hearing and their sense of touch.

A second important factor in this stage is that of conservation, which is the ability to understand that quantity does not change if the shape changes. In other words, if a short and wide glass of water is poured into a tall and thin glass. Children in this stage will perceive the taller glass as having more water due only because of it's height. This is due to the children's inability to understand *reversibility* and to focus on only one aspect of a stimulus (called cent ration), such as height, as opposed to understanding other aspects, such as glass width.

Developmental Stage and Age Characteristics Behaviours

Pre-operational Phase (2-4 years)	Increased use of verbal representation but speech is egocentric. The beginnings of symbolic rather than simple motor play. Transductive reasoning. Can think about something without the object being present by use of language.
Intuitive Phase (4-7 years)	Speech becomes more social, less egocentric. The child has an intuitive grasp of logical concepts in some areas. However, there is still a tendency to focus attention on

one aspect of an object while ignoring others. Concepts formed are crude and irreversible. Easy to believe in magical increase, decrease, disappearance. Reality not firm. Perceptions dominate judgment. In moral-ethical realm, the child is not able to show principles underlying best behaviour. Rules of a game not develop, only uses simple do's and don'ts imposed by authority.

Period of Concrete Operations (7-11 Years)

Concrete Operations Stage: Occurring between ages 7 and about 12, the third stage of cognitive development is marked by a gradual decrease in centristic thought and the increased ability to focus on more than one aspect of a stimulus. They can understand the concept of grouping, knowing that a small dog and a large dog are still both dogs, or that pennies, quarters, and dollar bills are part of the bigger concept of money.

They can only apply this new understanding to concrete objects (those they have actually experienced). In other words, imagined objects or those they have not seen, heard, or touched, continue to remain somewhat mystical to these children, and abstract thinking has yet to develop.

Period of Formal Operations (11-15 Years)

Formal Operations Stage: In the final stage of cognitive development (from age 12 and beyond), children begin to develop a more abstract view of the world. They are able to apply reversibility and conservation to both real and imagined situations. They also develop an increased understanding of the world and the idea of cause and effect. By the teenage years, they are able to develop their own theories about the world. This stage is achieved by most children, although failure to do so has been associated with lower intelligence.

Stages of Cognitive Growth

Ages 4 to 7 Months: Cognitive Development

During your baby's first four months, did you have doubts that she really understood much that was happening around her? This parental reaction is not surprising. After all, although you knew when she was comfortable and uncomfortable, she probably showed few signs of actually thinking. Now, as her memory and attention span increase, you'll start to see evidence that she's not only absorbing information but also applying it to her day-to-day activities.

Age 2 to 3 Years: Cognitive Development

That was a time when he learned about the world by touching, looking, manipulating and listening. Now the learning process has become more thoughtful. His grasp of language is increasing and he's beginning to form mental images for things, actions and concepts. He also can solve some problems in his head, performing mental trial-and-error instead of having to manipulate objects physically. And as his memory and intellectual abilities develop, he'll begin to understand simple time concepts.

Toddler also is starting to understand the relationship between objects. For instance, he'll be able to match similar shapes when you give him shape-sorting toys and simple jigsaw puzzles. He'll begin to recognize the purpose of numbers in counting objects, especially the number 2. And as his understanding of cause and effect develops, he'll become much more interested in winding up toys and turning lights and appliances on and off.

Age 3 to 4 Years: Cognitive Development

3-year-old will spend most of her waking hours questioning everything that happens around her. She loves to ask, "Why do I have to...?" and she'll pay close attention to your answers as long as they're simple and to the point. Don't feel that you have to explain your rules fully; she can't yet understand such reasoning and isn't interested in it anyway. If you try to have this kind of "serious" conversation, you'll quickly see her stare into space or turn her attention to more entertaining matters, like a toy across the room or a truck passing outside the window. Instead, telling her to do something "because it's good for you" or "so you don't get hurt" will make more sense to her than a detailed explanation.

Brain Growth

- Encourage playing with blocks and soft toys, which helps child develop eye-hand coordination, fine-motor skills and a sense of competence.
- Give consistent warm, physical contact - hugging, skin-to-skin, body-to-body contact to establish your toddler's sense of security and well-being.
- Be attentive to your child's rhythms and moods. Respond to her when she is upset as well as when she is happy. Be encouraging and supportive, with firm discipline as appropriate, but without yelling or hitting. Provide consistent guidelines.
- Talk or sing to child during dressing, bathing, feeding, playing, walking and driving, using adult talk. Speak slowly and give child time to respond. Try not to reply with "uh-huh" because child will recognize when you're not listening; instead, expand upon child's phrases.
- Be predictable; establish a pattern for mealtimes, naps and bedtime.

- Develop word associations by giving word labels to everyday objects and activities.

Age 4 to 5 Years: Cognitive Development

By age 4, the child is beginning to explore many basic concepts that will be taught in greater detail in school. For example, she now understands that the day is divided into morning, afternoon and night, and that there are different seasons. By the time she enters kindergarten she may know some days of the week, and that each day is measured in hours and minutes. She also may comprehend the essential ideas of counting, the alphabet, size relationships (big versus small) and the names of geometric shapes.

Activity of Child According to Age in Cognitive Growth

One-Year-Old Children

- They are curious.
- They point to objects that they want.
- They imitate animal sounds.
- They name familiar people and objects.
- They combine two words to form a basic sentence.
- They use the pronouns me and mine.
- They use "no" frequently.
- They name body parts and familiar pictures.
- They use objects for their intended purpose.
- They begin to include a second person in pretend play.
- Their attention span is short.
- They can hold a pencil and scribble.
- They are very active.
- Because of their developing imagination, they have trouble knowing what is real and what is pretend.

Two-Year-Old Children

- They follow simple directions.
- They use three or more words in combination.
- They express their feelings and wishes.
- They use objects to represent other objects.
- They still have a very limited attention span.
- They can memorize short rhymes.
- They join in simple songs.
- They begin to think about doing something before doing it.
- They have trouble making choices, but they want to make choices.

Three-Year-Old Children

- They can communicate their needs, ideas, and questions.
- Their attention span is a little longer so they can participate in group activities.
- Preschool children learn best by doing. They need a variety of activities. They need indoor and outdoor space. They need a balance between active and quiet play.

Four-Year-Old Children

- They are very talkative.
- They enjoy serious discussions.
- They ask lots of questions, including "how" and "why" questions.
- Their language includes silly words and profanity.
- Their classification skills and reasoning ability are developing.
- They should understand some basic concepts such as number, size, weight, colour, texture, distance, time, and position.

- [illegible]
- They follow complex directions
- [illegible]
- [illegible]
- [illegible]

31

Emotional Growth

Emotions means organize behaviour, energize behaviour and disrupt behaviour. It is a conscious process involving bodily changes. It adds to pleasure of everyday experience, serves as a motive to action and determine the characteristics pattern of adjustment of life. Child's emotions are first diffused and not very clear cut.

You are your child's first and favorite role model. You can send a positive message to her–that she is capable of doing many things. Start by being supportive. Take pleasure in child's accomplishments and let her know it.

Lover child and show your affection for her. Hug her, cuddle with her, read to her, talk to her throughout the day.

Encourage your child to try new things and to believe in her abilities. As she becomes a toddler, give her opportunities to play with other children her age. She will watch and imitate these new friends to learn new skills.

Needs

1. All children need to be comforted when they are upset.

Hold your child. Speak soothingly and calmly. She will let you know when she is feeling okay again.

2. Spend time with your child and help her explore her world and get to know the people in it.

3. Young children need consistent routines. Have a few routines and stick to them. This helps your child make sense of the world and become confident that events happen in an orderly fashion.

4. Be attuned to your child. Let her see you happy or sad when she is. She will learn that you can share the same emotions she has. This will help her learn to have empathy for others.

5. Children pass through many stages in social and emotional development. Some of their progress depends on nature (genetics) and some on nurture (the many loving and supportive things we do to help our children develop). Often, a child will temporarily slide back into a previous stage. This is only temporary and you will probably know of a recent upsetting event that caused this regression. For instance, your two-year-old starts asking for a bottle again. Maybe she has seen the attention a new baby nephew with a bottle is receiving from the family. With patience and love, your child will soon be back on track.

Stages of Emotional Growth

Age 0-12 Months

Your infant is fascinated by her immediate surroundings. She'll spend some months taking in information and learning how to deal with it in her own way. She is learning how to calm, comfort, and reassure herself. She is developing a sense of trust in those closest to her.

By about four months, your baby will begin to smile, laugh, and really enjoy being with others. It is so exciting to hear her laugh out loud, especially when you hear that first real "belly" laugh.

Infants are in love with life. They're also in love with their parents– the people they know will meet their every need. Your eight-month-old baby is learning to communicate with you about her needs. She will let you know when she's ready for play time, quiet time, and nap time.

By 10 months, your baby is the star of her world. She is developing confidence in her abilities and she needs for you to acknowledge them by showing your excitement. Let her lead your play. Observe and follow her lead. Her confidence will grow daily.

Age 1-2 Years

Your two-year-old, who once considered you her favourite playmate, is now beginning to enjoy playing near other children. She is watching and learning from them. She will sing and dance with others. She jealously guards her possessions. She is beginning to engage in very simple dramatic play involving the home. She has learned to imitate her mother's behaviour. She loves the word "no" and uses it often. She is confident in her actions and she can complete tasks. She dominates her world and when those around her don't do as she likes, she can be very stubborn. Avoid power struggles. They will leave both of you exhausted and unhappy. Offer choices instead. The choices you offer can be controlled by you. Set some common sense limits. Once you have set limits, be consistent in enforcing them.

Your two-year-old likes to watch other children play and may join briefly in their play, then withdraw to watch again. This is all very normal. She is learning about the world around her and the social skills she'll need to be a part of it, by watching others. This is also a great time to begin to teach your child to use her words to solve conflicts rather than hitting, or throwing a tantrum.

Children at this age can be easily distracted. Do not force her to keep on doing an activity when you can tell she has lost interest. You can try the activity again another day.

Age 2-3 Years

Three-year-old no longer hesitates when she sees a group of children at play. Instead, she jumps right in, ready to play, too. She loves pretend play. She has enough language to make herself understood and she is ready and eager to use it. She is learning that other people have feelings and she tries to be nice to everyone. She is even learning to wait for her turn. She wants to be everybody's friend. She is actually beginning to share. Three-year-olds will use "please" and "thank you" if they have heard it from you at home.

She's learning that it is okay to make a mistake. She is eager to please you and wants to do things right. Three-year-olds love to be praised and to show off all of their accomplishments. Give lots of hugs and encouragement! She loves it when you have time to play with her and she is even beginning to ask for your help when she needs it.

If you send your child to a preschool or to a child care programme, she may have problems with separation for a few weeks. She is so close to you that it will be hard for her to be away from you for so long. At this age, life is so interesting to children that it probably won't be long until she eagerly looks forward to being with her friends each day. If you do not send your child to preschool, consider taking her to a playgroup twice a week. The experience she will gain in playing with others will help prepare her for kindergarten.

Age 3-4 Years

Four-year-olds have strong likes and dislikes. They hate to lose games. They hate for things to be unfair.

They love fantasy play and reality-based play. They love simple board games. They love their parents and their teachers. They are trying to learn all they can about their parents. Often, your four-year-old will choose one parent to study and imitate and leave out the other. Later, she will decide to study the other parent and exclude the one she has just been totally absorbed with. Just give her time and she will pass through this stage and be loving and friendly to both of you again.

Four-year-olds are also very interested in their gender identity. This is one of the reasons they study each parent individually. They are establishing in their own minds what it means to be a boy or a girl. Your child may benefit from preschool or a playgroup this year. She'll develop the social and emotional skills she'll need to succeed in kindergarten.

Characteristics of Emotion

There are certain characteristics features of children's emotion.

1. Children's emotions are for short term and brief, it last for few minute.
2. Children's emotions are very intense.
3. Children's emotion arise in minor situation.
4. Children's emotions are transitory.
5. Children's emotions re not changeable.
6. Children's emotions appear frequently.
7. Children's emotions grows with increase in age.
8. Children's emotional responses are different.
9. Children's emotions are identified from the symptoms of behaviour.
10. Children's emotion change in strength.
11. Children's emotions are shows with expression change.

32

Individual Difference

Every individual takes birth on this earth with a kind of physiological and biological similarity. The process of development from birth to death is more or less alike in all individuals. Some common qualities found in almost all persons. Every person is endowed with a head, two hands, nose, ears etc. to make his living possible on this earth.

Therefore so many similarities there are also many dissimilarities among individuals. An individual has his own style of living his own personality and his own way of understanding the world. One thing must be clear that the differences found with man from man is quantitative not qualitative. This means physical, cognitive, moral and social traits are found in different quantities with different persons. Hence individual difference is of degree not of kind.

Individual Difference in Children

It is a common experience with almost all parents and teachers that they think of children of the same age as being alike and consequently except similar behaviour from them or they except what work with one child with automatically work with another child. But it should be remembered that though the pattern of development is similar for all children, the way and rate of development differs. Some children develop in a smooth, gradual, step-by-step fashion, while others move in spruts. Some show slight swings. While others show wide ones. All children do not therefore, reach the same point of development at the same age. In other words all children of the same age cannot be expected to behave in the same way. child from a socially backward environment cannot display the same ability in reading and writing as a child coming from an educationally conscious environment. Another example is that a child reared up in a authoritarian control shows difference n his sociality from a child reared up in a democratic set up. A particular joke make appear hilarious for one child, while the other child may consider it boring or stupid.

It is provided that children follow a pattern of development that is characterize their and controlled by their own unique combination of hereditary endowment and environmental factors. This display a certain consistency of development. For example children who are tall at one age are tall a other ages. Likewise those who are short remain short. Similarity children with accelerated mental growth continue to be accelerated and who are mentally deficient lack the ability to catch up, rather they are likely to become more and more retarded as they grow older. Experiment of Bayley, an America psychologist prove that the developmental processes of children are relatively similar at first, but around 6 years of age individual difference begins to appear.

Type of Individual Difference

Individual difference is not limited to any person, place or time. It is universal and a law of nature. Psychologist have conducted experiments on its nature and extent to shed light on its educational implications. Generally children is a class or school come from almost all walks of life with different status, heredity, sex, and caste etc. Again there is no restriction on admission of students in our schools. Just pay the frees and get admitted. This tendency make individual difference more prominent and vivid in our country.

Individual differences can broadly be divided into two types:

1. Inter individual difference.
2. Intra individual difference.

When abilities, interest and personality of individual difference that is called inter-individual difference.

But when difference from one ability to another within ones own self is marked. It is known as intra-individual difference. This is the difference within the individual which is otherwise known ad difference in traits.

Causes of Individual Difference

Dobzhansky once said "every person is indeed biologically and genetically different from every other". Again environmental influences of two person may never be the same, even not in case of identical twins. Hence it is proved that individual difference is caused by both internal and external factors. This makes the pattern of development different for every child, even though major aspects of this pattern is similar.

Psychologists view that there are various causes of individual difference. Heredity and environment are the most fundamental of them. But there was quite a controversy raised regarding their relative importance. One school of thought claimed heredity to be the foremost manipulator of human personality. Whereas some other psychologists were of the view that environment plays the most important role in building personality. Galton described it as the controversy between nature and nature. Some other factors responsible for human variations are sex, race, nationality, physique, age and personality etc.

Heredity

Heredity means the native inborn qualities in terms of abilities, capacities and aptitude with which each individual starts the business of life. Psychologists believed that variation in genes causes individual difference.

Environment

Psychologist and sociologists have shed light on the influence of social and cultural surroundings on individual difference among men. Various experiments shows on animals it has been proved that child's mental ability is affected by per natal and post-natal environments. Environments, nutrition of the mother, diseases she suffers from and drugs, she is habituated with during pregnancy, affects the intellectual development of the infant before birth. Apart from all these a number of social factors determines the level and degree of intelligence of the human being.

Intelligence

It is complex and controversial topic in psychology. It is one of those factors that influence human behaviour. According to T.P. Nunn for all the times "you" and "I" are two separate personalities. As the course of two rivers can never be the same. Likewise two individuals cannot show identical behaviour. It is clear from his opinion that intelligence cause individual difference among persons.

Need of Education for Individual Difference

Though psychologists very often discuss about the individual difference among children, our educational system and specially teachers seem not to take it so seriously. Our educational practice is still planned as if pupils are all of one piece, more or less equally capable of profiting by classroom teaching. Difference in mental growth, learning, interest, aptitudes and other competencies are not fully taken into consideration to draw the best possible result out of it.

It is an established fact that children have different goals, different interests, different emotional problems and different abilities. The content, curriculum, method, programmes and patterns of educational activity should respond to the varying needs, interest, and abilities of children. Here arises a problem for teachers when on one hand they have a school work, that is planned on group basis and on the other hand every individual child is to be dealt with according to his caliber.

The first task of a teacher in a class is to know and study individual difference among his pupils. He may make an I.Q. test and grade the students into various grades. Students with an I.Q. of 130 are genius and the teachers, responsibility is to offer encouragement and guidance and leave the rest to pupil. But with a pupil whose I.Q. is 70 or less, He has to be very patient. He has to repeat explanation, approach the topic of teaching and study from various angles and review his work, and still the pupil may not be able to comprehend or give correct answer.

An intimate knowledge of individual difference among children will go a long way to way to make education child centred, realistic and positive. Modern schools should try to adjust themselves to the pupil rather than excepting the pupil to adjust himself to the school. Without this all educational efforts will become ineffective. Every pupil should be allowed to grow and develop at his own rate.

If we have to classify the students into group, that would enhance their learning by giving proper attention to their individual difference, then what should be the basis of classification is a matter of discussion. There are a large number of classification such as mental age, intelligence quotient, average attainment in all subjects, average marks in important subjects, achievement test score, teacher's rating of pupil ability, physical or social maturity etc. In primary or elementary schools classification may be based on I.Q. but in past primary classes students may be grouped by achievement in different subjects. In large schools retarded and slow learners should be taught in special classes and suitable programmer should be devised for them. There may be physical defects in students like defects in hearing and seeing. This could be detected by proper medical check up. Our promotion system does not respond in a positive way to individual difference in children.

Though there is little doubt that studying individual difference is very important in educational system, still then it is very difficult to classify pupils on their basis. Some most important requirements in this regard are greater flexibility of organization, cooperation between teachers and pupils and above all a deep interest in each and every individual student by the teacher.

33

Personality

Introduction

Personality is constituted within the person. It develops in certain directions. Apart from its impact on our physical activities, personality also influences our inner traits and life style. As a result the inner personality of an individual becomes more important than his outward appearance.

Personality is the sum total of inherited and acquired traits, desires, inspiration and nature.

Personality is determined by the interaction of temperament traits with the environment. Each person (including your child) comes with a factory installed wiring. How your child is wired can determine whether they will be easy or difficult to raise. How well their temperament fits with the environment and how well they are received by the people in the environment will determine how a child sees himself and others.

Definition

Define personality in terms of social stimulus value, by which an individual can influence other persons he meets in his own way.

According to R.B. Cattle, "personality is that which permits a prediction of what a person will do in a given situation.

Personality is always dynamic and changing in nature. It is neither static nor rigid. It expresses and manifests itself differently in various circumstances.

Personality is a product of actions and their reaction. It is always active. It is never passive or static.

Concept

An individual's personality is the complex of mental characteristics that makes them unique from other people. It includes all of the patterns of thought and emotions that cause us to do and say things in particular ways. At a basic level, personality is expressed through our temperament or emotional tone. However, personality also colours our values, beliefs, and expectations. There are many potential factors that are involved in shaping a personality. These factors are usually seen as coming from heredity and the environment. Research by psychologists over the last several decades has increasingly pointed to hereditary factors being more important, especially for basic personality traits such as emotional tone. However, the acquisition of values, beliefs, and expectations seem to be due more to socialization and unique experiences, especially during childhood.

Factors Affecting Personality

Personality is always developing and enlarging. Its development start from the birth of a child till the end of his life. So many inner and outside factors are responsible for its dynamic nature. These are the factors which influence the personality growth: heredity, environment, family, school, teacher, failure, society, culture etc.

Some hereditary factors that contribute to personality development do so as a result of interactions with the particular social environment in which people live. For instance, your genetically inherited physical and mental capabilities have an impact on how others see you and, subsequently, how you see yourself. If you have poor motor skills that prevent you from throwing a ball straight and if you regularly get bad grades in school, you will very likely be labeled by your teachers, friends, and relatives as someone who is inadequate or a failure to some degree. This can become a self-fulfilling prophesy as you increasingly perceive yourself in this way and become more pessimistic about your capabilities and your future. Likewise, your health and physical appearance are likely to be very important in your personality development. You may be frail or robust. You may have a learning disability. You may be slender in a culture that considers obesity attractive or vice versa. These largely hereditary factors are likely to cause you to feel that you are nice-looking, ugly, or just adequate. Likewise, skin colour, gender, and sexual orientation are likely to have a major impact on how you perceive yourself. Whether you are accepted by others as being normal or abnormal can lead you to think and act in a socially acceptable or marginal and even deviant way.

There are many potential environmental influences that help to shape personality. Child rearing practices are especially critical. In North America, children are usually raised in ways that encourage them to become self-reliant and independent. Children are often allowed to act somewhat like equals to their parents. For instance, they are included in making decisions about what type of food and entertainment the family will have on a night out. Children are given allowances and small jobs around the house to teach them how to be responsible for themselves. In contrast, children in China are usually encouraged to think and act as a member of their family and to suppress their own wishes when they are in conflict with the needs of the family. Independence and self-reliance are viewed as an indication of family failure and are discouraged. It is not surprising that Chinese children traditionally have not been allowed to act as equals to their parents.

Despite significant differences in child rearing practices around the world, there are some similarities. Boys and girls are socialized differently to some extent in all societies. They receive different messages from their parents and other adults as to what is appropriate for them to do in life. They are encouraged to prepare for their future in jobs fitting their gender. Boys are more often allowed freedom to experiment and to participate in physically risky activities. Girls are encouraged to learn how to do domestic chores and to participate in child rearing by baby-sitting. If children do not follow these traditional paths, they are often labeled as marginal or even deviant—girls may be called "tomboys" and boys may be ridiculed for being "effeminate."

There are always unique situations and interpersonal events that help to shape our personalities. Such things as having alcoholic parents, being seriously injured in a car accident, or being raped can leave mental scars that make us fearful and less trusting. If you are an only child, you don't have to learn how to compromise as much as children who have several siblings. Chance meetings and actions may have a major impact on the rest of our lives and affect our personalities. For instance, being accepted for admission to a prestigious university or being in the right place at the right time to meet the person who will become your spouse or life partner can significantly alter the course of the rest of your life. Similarly, being drafted into the military during wartime, learning that you were adopted, or personally witnessing a tragic event, such as the destruction of the World Trade Center towers in New York, can change your basic perspective.

Types of Personality

The concept of national personality types primarily had its origins in anthropology with the research of Ruth Benedict beginning in the 1920's. She believed that personality was almost entirely learned. She said that normal people acquire a distinct *ethos*, or culturally specific personality pattern, during the process of being uncultivated as children. Benedict went on to say that our cultural personality patterns are assumed to be "natural" by us and other personality patterns are viewed as being "unnatural" and deviant. She said that such feelings are characteristic of all people in all cultures because we are ethnocentric. Benedict compared the typical personalities of the 19th century North American Plains Indians with those of the farming Pueblo Indians of the American Southwest. She said that the bison hunting Plains Indians had personalities that could be typified as being aggressive, prone to violence, and seeking extreme emotional states. In contrast, she said that the typical Pueblo Indian was just the opposite—peaceful, non-aggressive, and sober in personality.

Benedict's views were especially popular in the 1930's among early feminists such as her student Margaret Mead. This was because if personality is entirely learned, it means that feminine and masculine personality traits are not biologically hard-wired in. In other words, culture rather than genes, makes women nurturing towards children and passive in response to men. Likewise, culture makes men aggressive and domineering. If this is true, these stereotypical behaviours can be altered and even reversed. Mead carried out ethnographic field work among the Polynesian peoples of the South Pacific to find examples of societies in which femininity and masculinity have very different and even opposite characteristics from those found in the Western World. She also found in Samoa, a relaxed adolescence in which sex is talked about freely by boys and girls rather than hidden or suppressed.

Most anthropologists today believe that Benedict and her students went too far in their assertions about the influence of culture on personality formation and in discounting heredity. They also tended to over simplify by defining people who did not share all of the traits of the "national personality type" as being deviants. It is more accurate to see the members of a society as having a range of personality types.

Modal Personality: This is the most common personality type within a society. In reality, there is usually a range of normal personality types within each society.

In the early 1950's, David Riesman proposed that there are three common types of modal personality that occur around the world. He called them tradition oriented, inner-directed, and other directed personalities.

1. Tradition-oriented Personality is one that places a strong emphasis on doing things the same way that they have always been done. Individuals with this sort of personality are less likely to try new things and to seek new experiences.

2. Inner-directed Personalities are guilt oriented. That is to say, their behaviour is strongly controlled by their conscience. As a result, there is little need for police to make sure that they obey the law. These individuals monitor themselves. If they break the law, they are likely to turn themselves in for punishment.

3. Other-directed Personalities have ambiguous feelings about right and wrong. When they deviate from a societal norm, they usually don't feel guilty. However, if they are caught in the act or exposed publicly, they are likely to feel shame.

Advocates of Riesman's concept of three modal personalities suggest that the tradition-oriented personality is most common in small-scale societies and in some sub-cultures of large-scale ones. Inner-directed personalities are said to be more common in some large-scale societies, especially ones that are culturally homogeneous. In contrast, the other-directed personality is likely to be found in culturally diverse large-scale societies in which there is not a uniformity in socialization processes and there is considerable anonymity for city dwellers.

Theories of Personality

The true nature of personality, different theories have been advocated by psychologist. Some important theories are: Type theory, Trait theory and Psychoanalytic theory.

Classification

The famous psychologist Sigmund Freud has classified personality into three types. This is based on his theory of psycho- sexual development of child. Human development n each of its stage is influenced by his instincts. The classification is discussed below:

1. Oral erotic type sex instinct during babyhood is located at mouth is a kind of pleasure seeking and life maintaining energy focused on certain object and goals. This experience in infancy produced two types of personality in future: They are (i) oral passive type. (ii) oral sadistic type.

2. **Theanal Type:** The child during this stage expresses his satisfaction or dissatisfaction through anal expulsion or anal manipulation. On the influence of this stage a person in future shows disobedience, miserly and indiscipline behaviour.

3. **Phallic Type:** This stage is characterized by pleasant and entertaining behavior. Such people are self centred and try to attract others towards their own way. They like to show themselves and get pleasure from this.

34

Learning Process

Introduction

The layman's idea about learning is that it is acquisition of knowledge. Typically it is supposed that a man or animal had some experience–either because, the environment put some sensory information into one of its senses or it tried out some form of action and observed its consequence. This experience which he acquires guides him in his behaviours. He modified his behaviour in the light of his past experience, so that he can respond correctly to his environment. Hence his learning ultimately leads to the modification of his behaviour. That is why psychologists define learning as modification of behaviour.

Definition

Man learns new methods and skills to successfully do, think, reason and adjust to any forthcoming problems. Learning is associated with acquisition of new behaviour or modification of old behaviour. Psychologist from their own viewpoints have defined learning in various ways.

While a student wants to learn more and more new ideas, a teacher tries to adopt a novel method of teaching.

According to skinner learning is not acquiring knowledge or skill by mere mechanical repetitions. It is a process in which the learner organizes different elements and experiences to reach a particular goal.

According to the Hilgard learning refers to the change in subject's behaviour to a given situation brought about by is repeated experiences in that situation, provided that the behaviour change cannot be explained on the basis of native response tendencies, maturation or temporary states of the subject.

According to Kinglay and Gray learning is the process by which an organism in satisfying its motivation adopts and adjusts its behaviour in order to over come obstacles or barriers.

According to Eason learning includes changes in behaviour that are determined primarily by the individuals interaction with his environment.

According to Cronback learning is shown by a change in behaviour as a result of experience.

According to Garret learning is an organization of behaviour. It is the activity by virtue of which we organize our responses with new habits.

According to Murphy learning is an a modification of both behaviour and the way of perceiving.

Nature of Learning

Man not only learn but also train the lower animal. What learning does for a human child and how it affects his lifestyle is clear from the discussion below:

1. Learning is modification of behaviour.
2. Learning helps to reach the goal.
3. Learning creates interest to know new things.
4. Environmental influence bring difference in learning.

5. Learning is problem solving activity.
6. Learning is a master of habits.
7. Learning is an automatic process.
8. Learning is not knowledge about subjects.
9. Learning may be correct or incorrect.
10. Learning occurs both in formal and informal situation.
11. Higher learning depends upon capacity of individual and complexity of learning material.
12. Learning a function of maturation.
13. Learning is dependent on nervous system.
14. Learning a self acting process.

Characteristics of Learning

Educational psychology has given a detail of the characteristics of learning processes. They are:

1. Learning is a continuous change in behaviour. It is a life long process.
2. It is comprehensive. It affects every aspects of human life.
3. Learning is physically, emotionally, and cognitively attached with the whole of the person.
4. Learning brings change in the discipline of behaviour.
5. Learning is development.
6. Learning is encouragement. Sometimes it becomes more influential motivator than some direct stimulus such as reinforcement and some indirect stimulus such as fear of punishment.
7. Learning is always directed towards a goal, and all the behaviour of the learner are modified in such a way that he may reach that goal.
8. Learning and interest are linked with each other. An individual leans better when he becomes interested in that particular subjects.

9. Learning depends upon motivation and readiness. In many case physical maturation is required before learning.

10. The goals and motives sometimes direct our behaviour to be organized in a certain manner. When that organized behaviour becomes ale to reach the goal, it becomes permanent.

11. Trial and error experience and insightful learning experience brings change in the mode of reaction to the environment.

12. In the process of solving the problem the individual reacts to his environment. The stamped in reactions become habitual and in the end emerges as a learned material.

Learning and Maturation

Learning and maturation are interrelated. But they are distinguishable. Maturation signifies the process of growth and development. It occurs in the absence of any sort of habits, training or stimulus. On the other hand learning is the modification of behaviour which is result of experience and training.

Significant condition in learning

The process of learning is affected by certain condition. A knowledge of these conditions is essential for every teacher and parents, because by manipulating these conditions they can bring a required change in the behavior of the child. Some of the important conditions are discussed below:

1. Readiness
2. Motivation
3. Interest
4. Attention
5. Drill or practice
6. Fatigue and boredom
7. Intelligence

8. Aptitude
9. Attitude
10. Emotional factors
11. Family and cultural expectancies

Learning by doing and Playing

Learning is associated with playing or merry making, it becomes more effective. It arouses interest in them to learn. Teaching should not be only giving lectures to the students. They become bored by that. Secondly, if while learning a skill the learner does the work with his own hands he masters it without much effort. Modern methods of teaching gives stress upon play way method and discards the conventional reciting in classroom method. Now the classrooms have turned into play ground.

Factors Affecting Learning

Learning is a process, this process depends upon a number of factors. If we categorizes the factors upon which this process is based on, we will find three main directions. They are:

1. The internal condition of the learner—such as capacity, motivation, age, sex difference, experiences etc.

2. Nature of the subject to be learnt—such as span or range of learning, complexity or simplicity of learning materials etc.

3. Methods of learning—such as memorization, analysis, drilling, recitation etc.

35

Language Growth

Language is a communication form. It is a media by which distinguishes baby from animal. Child feel more secure when he gets command over language. It is a communication skill which display the behaviour. Language is a form of speech by which one can understand feeling of others. Speech is a media between two person which convey the meaning. Speech means utteration or pronounciation of words which is known as language. Speech is one type of behavior that helps the child to move from world of socialized relationship. Child with good language able establish better social relationship. Child expresses his feeling, thought and attitudes more freely. Speech is a complex process. Language is closely associated with corresponding developments in speech organs, mouth development and ability of the child to associate sounds with meaningful events, objects and persons.

Language has two different aspects:

1. Language production.
2. Language comprehension.

The chart below presents typical language development.

Causes of Disorder in Language Growth

Language disorders may be caused by:

- Hearing loss
- Ear infections
- Neurological (brain or nerve) disorders

- Brain or head injury
- Mental retardation (developmental delay)
- Stroke
- Viral infections
- Physical problems such as cleft lip or cleft palate
- Autism
- Cerebral palsy
- Learning disabilities

Defective Language

Speech defects arise either due to malformation of the speech organ or due to emotional disturbances. Following are the some common defective speech:

1. Lisping: It is structured of letter sound substitution, children while pronounce "simple simon" pronounce "thimple thimon" or "red rose" called as "wed wose". This happens due to defective teeth, jaw, tongue or fascination for using baby speech. Children due one or other reason substitute the for "s", "Z", "w" for "r" and so on. After their permanent teeth appear, their lisping decreases. In rare cases due to organic defects or space between teeth lisping may be occur.

2. Stammering: Stammering is a type of stuttering means prolongation of the sound of the opening letter of a word i.e. b....... bath. Stammering occurs when a child cannot get a word out. Some children have problems with consonants and not in another.

3. Stuttering: It is a kind of speech defect and also repetitive speech, it occurs due to failure of speech muscle to co-ordinate. It appears that the person dose not know suddenly what to say, often accompanied by stammering. There is check of speech followed by sudden speech which then is followed by no speech and so on. It appears due to poor vocabulary, overprotective parents, dominant and over anxious parents. These factors are responsible for stuttering. It is a form of speech impediment which is common in pre-school children. The most complicated task the child faces during preschool year is the process of learning to talk. Stuttering disappears if the parents do not make an issues of it and if they let the child finish his utterance without correcting him, or calling attention to his difficulties interrupting. It can be treated with build sense of security and self-confidence.

4. Slurring: Not clear speech in child called slurring. It occurs due to inactivity of the lips, paralysis of vocal organs, timidity, excitement or fear for the strangers. It mostly appears during post school years. Slurring is corrected if the child opens his mouth while speaking so that sounds can come outside. They speak so fast that no body can understand what they say.

5. Cluttering: It is a jumping speech defects. IT a rapid, confused and jumbled type of speech. It is just like stuttering. But the more one tries to control it, the more of it you shall have. Children whose speech development has been delayed give evidence of cluttering.

Factors Affecting Language Development

Following are some factors which influenced the speech and language development.

Health

The child suffers from severe and prolonged illness during the first two years of life, language development is impaired. Illness not only delays the development of speech organs but isolation and seclusions confines communication with adults concurrently.

Intelligence

Intelligence play a vital role in language development. Babbling at an early age are better predictor of child's intelligence. Children of high intelligence show better linguistic competence both in vocabulary, length of sentences uttered and correctness of sentence structure.

Socio Economic Condition of Family

Those children from high socio economic status talk faster, talk better than the poor children. Lower group of children suffer from listening elaborative language, suffer from under and over stimulation, and commit more articulation errors. The relationship between socio- economic condition and language ability is well established and the gap in language competence and production becomes more between high and low socio-economic groups as age advances.

Sex

Boys are faster then the girls in learning to talk. Compared to girls the length of sentence uttered by boys is less. The comprehension vocabulary is also small in case of boys. Boys commit more grammatical errors and their pronunciation is less accurate. Sex difference in favour of girls remain and become quite pounced with every increase in age.

Family Relationship

A healthy stimulating environment facilitates language development, particularly the relationship between mother and child. Children reared in institutions are slow in learning to talk, and remain retarded in language development throughout their lives. This happens primarily because of lack of adequate adult contact and personal relationship in the institution.

Twins

Twins and triplets are slower to learn the language than the single child. Their vocabulary skill is so faster than the twins.

Bilingual Homes

In bilingual homes the child face several problems to the language because the learn more than two languages at a time so it is very difficult to child remember the two or three languages at a time.

reasoned in language development throughout [illegible] This [illegible] [illegible] [illegible] [illegible] and [illegible] [illegible]

Notes

[illegible]

Summary

[illegible]

36

Social Growth

Socialization is the process of presenting alternate channels for individual behaviour together with positive and negative sanctions emphasizes the influence social groups, formal and informal upon the personality of the individual. It involves three processes:

1. Child behaves according to the norms of his own group.

2. Child plays appropriate sex roles and other roles and defined by the group, parents, and children etc.

3. Child develops proper social attitudes.

Social development is a slow process. There are periods of development. It is quite rapid at first. Social development follows a pattern. Social development is predictable.

During the first three years of life, your child will develop crucial social abilities, learn to give and accept love, to be confident and secure, to show empathy, to be curious and persistent—all abilities that will enable your child to learn, relate well to others and lead a happy and productive life. This is an exciting period in your child's life!

Each child grows and develops differently. This gives you general information about what a child from birth to age five might be doing at a certain age.

Social Growth

2-4 Weeks: Raises head momentarily when prone. Fixes on human face and follows with eyes. Responds to parent's face and voice, smiles spontaneously. Responds to sound by blinking, crying, quieting, changing respiration or showing startle response. Has flexed posture; moves all extremities. Can sleep for three or four hours at a time; can stay awake for one hour. Can be consoled most of the time by being spoken to or held.

2 Months: Grasps rattle placed in hand. Social smiles, smiles responsively. Coos and reciprocal vocalization. Shows interest in visual and auditory stimuli. Demonstrates social interaction, follows moving person with eyes. When prone, lifts head, neck and upper chest with support of forearms. Some head control in upright position.

4 Months: Holds head high, raises body on hands when prone, sits when supported. Controls head well. Rolls prone to supine. Plays with hands, holds rattle, reaches for objects, holds own hands. Looks at mobile, arms active. Follows object 180 degrees. Smiles, coos, laughs, babbles; initiates social contact, turns to voice. May sleep at least six hours. Able to comfort self, e.g., fall asleep by self

6 Months: Rolls from front to back; sits with support. Bears weight, stands with support. Transfers objects hand to hand. Turns to sound and voice; may show stranger anxiety. Raking hand pattern; grasps and mouths objects. Vocalizes single consonants ("dada", "baba"); may imitate sounds of speech. Babbles reciprocally; reacts socially by smiling in response to someone else's smile. Shows recognition of parents; shows interest in toys. Starts to self-feed. First tooth may erupt.

9 Months: Sits independently. Reaches for objects with one hand. Crawls, creeps or scoots on bottom.

Pulls to stand, stands holding on. Inferior pincer grasp, pokes with index. Inferior pincer grasp, pokes with index finger. Bangs, throws and drops objects. Finger feeds, starts to use cup. Imitates vocalizations; babbles. May say "dada" and "mama" nonspecifically. Responds to own name. Understands a few words, e.g., "no-no," "bye-bye" – combines syllables. Can sleep through the night. May show stranger anxiety. Enjoys interactive games, e.g., peek-a-boo and pat-a-cake. Turns toward sound with eyes and head movement.

12 Months: Pulls to stand, stands alone, cruises, may take a few steps alone Has precise pincer grasp. Points; indicates wants. Has vocabulary of one to three words; uses "mama" and "dada" correctly. Recognizes caregiver's voice. Obeys simple requests; waves "bye-bye". Feeds self; drinks from a cup. Actively looks for hidden or dropped objects Shows emotions (fear, anxiety, affection) imitates.

15 Months: Walks alone, bends over, may run. Crawls up stairs. Stacks two blocks. Can point to one or more body parts. Feeds self with fingers, drinks from cup. Understands simple commands. Listens to a story. Has vocabulary of three to six words Indicates wants by pointing or grunting Imitates activity. Can remove some clothing.

18 Months: Likes to climb and run, walks backwards; climbs into chair, sits in chair Throws/kicks ball; stacks three or four blocks. Has a vocabulary of 15-20 words, uses two word phrases, imitates words. Uses a spoon and cup, can remove clothing. Listens to a story, looking at pictures and naming objects. Plays with toys appropriately, e.g., pulls a pull toy, cuddles a doll. Answers simple questions by pointing, follows simple directions. Scribbles spontaneously, imitates crayon strokes. Dumps object from bottle without demonstration. Shows affection, hugs and kisses

24 Months: Climbs up and down steps holding on with one hand. Jumps, runs, throws overhand. Stands on one foot with little support. Can stack five or six blocks. Has a vocabulary of 50+ words, two word phrases, understands pronouns. Speech should be intelligible to parents. Parallel play dominant. Possessive with toys. Can follow two-step commands, can name some body parts. Makes or imitates horizontal and circular strokes with crayon. Imitates adults. Increasing attention span Separation anxiety from parents. Brushes teeth with help, puts on clothing, washes hands.

3 Years: Jumps in place, kicks a ball, balances on one foot, stacks blocks. Rides a tricycle. Alternates feet ascending stairs. Knows name, age and gender. Copies circle and cross, visually discriminates colors. Has some self care skills, e.g., feeding and dressing self. Demonstrates speech that is mostly intelligible. Pretend play well developed Can follow directions Names colours.

4 Years: Hops, jumps forward, alternates feet when climbing stairs, balances on each foot, climbs. Rides a tricycle. Builds tower of 10 or more cubes, plays board/ card games. Throws overhand Ability to cut and paste. Draws a person with two or three parts; copies circle, cross and square. Can sing a song. Can talk about daily activities. Can distinguish fantasy from reality. Make believe play, imaginary playmates. Puts away own toys. Dresses and undresses self, brushes teeth with no help.

5 Years: Dresses self without help, ties shoelaces. Balances on each foot, heel-to-toe walk, can count on fingers Knows own address and phone number Recognizes colors and common shapes. Copies simple shapes (e.g., triangle or square), able to print a few letters and numbers. Draws a person with head, body, arm and legs. Speaks in phrases that are understood by others. Plays make believe and dress up. Plays and shares with others Understands opposites Recalls parts of stories.

Factors Relates to Social Development

1. Home: It is the first place which influence on the socialization of the child. The culture of the home, language of family members, the behaviours displayed by parents and elders slowly but surely become a part of the child's personality and socialization. So these influence the socialization.

2. Socio-economic Status: The child from low economic status face a lot of problems in his day to day life. A poor child cannot adjust with a high economic status child.

3. Relationship: It also play a vital role in social development. Parental relationship, children relationship, father–son and mother–daughter relationship which influence the social life.

4. Culture: It is powerful socializing agent in the life of an individual. Ancient society differ from modern society. A good culture makes a individual perfect but a bad culture makes a child delinquent.

5. Peer groups: Child behaviour influenced by peer group, they give approval and attention, affection and child imitate the behaviour of the peer groups.

6. Adult: Child influenced by adults ,when he enter to school he learn negative thing from senior and follow the attitude of the senior child.

7. Twins: They spend maximum time together, have more interests in common in outside companionships as compared to other siblings. They imitate each other and display same feeling.

8. Family Size: Small family secure greater economic advantage they do produce problems of over protection and occasional tensions in the child. Joint family provide less economic advantage.

9. Education and Occupation of Parents: They provide models for observation and imitation. Working both of parent effects on child development.

10. Urbanization and Modernization: It provide greater stimulation at the same time greater diversion for undesirable habits in children.

SECTION-D
HOME SCIENCE

37

Home Science and its Application

Introduction

Home Science not only helps in leading a better family life but also presents itself as a potential source of numerous career opportunities. You should surely be interested in finding out the usefulness of this subject in your daily lives.

(a) Home Science in Everyday Life

Home Science helps to meet the challenges of daily life with confident. It provides basic information required to make rational decision at home and outside. It equips one for caring for home, family, and for pursuing a career, to be a competent homemakers in today's world, you need a wide range of skills. The knowledge of Home Science enables one to develop these skills. These have a tremendous practical application in day-to-day life.

Study of Home Science helps one to acquire better individual understanding. Home Science students learn to identify and manage their houses. They acquire the skills needed to meet the basic needs of life in a family. Hence they are capable of taking care of food, clothing, shelter, education and health of all family members to a great extent.

(b) Home Science Supplementing Family

You have already learnt the need and importance of supplementing family income. There are so many ways of supplementing family income through skills learnt in Home Science.

(i) Offering Tuitions: Home Science is both applied science as well as art. You get a wide range of knowledge through its study. You also get to know the cognitive achievements of different developmental stages with this background you can successfully offer tuition for small children doing free time and thereby supplement family income.

(ii) Child Care: This subject provides you enough knowledge about needs and care of young children. During free hours, you can look after a few children on else offer your services to any nearby day care center on preparatory school and earn money.

(iii) Selling of Food Items: You have learnt to prepare various sweets, baking, you can demonstrate the preparation of sweets to a willing group of your neighbours and sell your prepared items as well. If you own an oven you can earn money by baking cakes on order.

(iv) Utilizing Skills of Rangoli: Flavour arrangement and clearing metal etc. Student get free time during summer vacations. You can supplement income by conducting summer classes on flower arrangement and floor decorative clearing and polishing of metal (gold, silver, brass) to make same money.

(v) Selling Handicraft Items: The skills of dyeing and block prinking can be used in supplementing family income. Articles like dupattas, mafeler, sarees, bed sheets etc. can be prepared using these techniques. Later these items can be sold during festive occasions like Diwali Mela etc.

Tailoring, stiching of dresses, embroidery, knitting of woollen garments to create beautiful utility to supplement income. Home Science helps one to increase money income and real income.

(c) Self Employment – Through Home

There is a common saying "look at the forest not the trees". It indicates that one must broaden one's knowledge, experience, observation and interests. Home Science is an applied course which enriches students with varied knowledge to develop skills.

Skills Required	*Opportunities for Self Employment*
Child Caring	Running Creche/day care center
Skills	Running play school

Creches, day care centers, pre-nursery and play schools can now be seen in almost all localities, Home Science student need to further develop their skills. The employment opportunities is connected with cooking skills are listed in the table below:

Skills Required	*Opportunities for self Employment*
Cooking and Calinary	Owning a bakery Contract catering services Mobile Catering Van Organizing hobby classes

(d) Home Science Related Careers

Home Science related to many vocations and offers varied opportunities in career today. These career are exciting relevant and much in demand. Below diagram shows the vocations relating to Home Science.

Institutions Providing Education and Training to Home Science

Both governments and non-government institutions are to provide teaching and knowledge in Home Science related field, to train further and refine the skills needed for the desired vocation and career.

Home Science Colleges

Almost all university offer Bachelor and Master Degree in Home Science studies. Master Degree are generally offered in areas namely Food and Nutrition, Resources Management, Child development, Textile designing and extension education. Some Home Science colleges also offer degree/diploma in Dietetics and public health nutrition. For becoming a university lecturer all students are required to qualify National eligibility test for lecturership conducted by University Grant Commission (UGC). Minimum requirement for lecturership is M.Sc. in this subject. One can also opt. For research work in the specialized field.

Institutes Providing Certificate Courses

Food craft institute, Fashion Technology institute, Hotel Management Institute offer certificate and diploma courses in different field of Home Science related studies. Facilities are also available for studying apparel Marketing and Merchandising, Public Relation, Personal Management etc. The duration for such courses ranges from 6 months to 4 years. The eligibility for these courses varies. Competitive entrances examination and Class XII Board results are the basic criterion of entry into the above courses.

Industrial Training Institute

Different states run these institutes to provide vocational training to youth to make themselves relevant. Diploma course in tailoring, dress designing, handicrafts, food preservation and food craft resources are run by government and non-government agencies. Polytechniques offers also diploma studies and courses are more expensive in polytechniques.

Various institutions providing distance education,

courses, who can not pursue their studies on regular basis. IGNOU also offer a variety of distance learning courses.

Bibliography

USDA/FSIS, *Food Borne Illness: What Consumers Need to Know*, September 1998.

Baldwin, A.L. (1955), *Behaviour and Development in Childhood*, New York.

Bowlby, J. (1951), *Maternal Care and Child Health.*

Partnership for Food Safety Education (1997). *Foodborne Illness. A Constant Challenge.*

Partnership for Food Safety Education (1997). *Four Simple Steps to Fight Back.*

Bayley, N. (1975), *On the Growth of Intelligence*, American Psychologist.

Ericson, E. (1950), *Childhood and Society*, New York.

Hurlock, E. (1972), *Child Development*, Tokyo.

Kohlberg, L. (1968), Early Education, a Cognitive Development View, Child Development.

Lenneberg, E.H. (1967), *Biological Function of Language.*

Panda, K.C. (1978), *Elements of Child Development.*

Dash, B.N. (1988), *Elements of Educational Psychology.*

Prem Lata Mallick, 1981, *Elements of Home Science.*

Index